getting baked

getting baked

Everything You Need to Know about

Hemp, CBD, and Medicinal Gardening

By Barb Webb

Published in the United States by Viva Editions, an imprint of Start Midnight, LLC, 221 River Street, Ninth Floor, Hoboken, New Jersey, 07030.

Printed in the United States
Cover design: Jennifer Do
Cover image: Shutterstock
Text design: Frank Wiedemann

First Edition.
10 9 8 7 6 5 4 3 2 1

Trade paper ISBN: 978-1-63228-071-8
E-book ISBN: 978-1-63228-127-2

To all the herbalists who designed the maps for navigating the natural path, I'm indebted to your wise teachings. To my husband and my children who always endure my quirks during the book writing process and constantly lift me up with their unconditional support and love, to my mermaid pirate sock soul sister who graciously volunteered as tribute to be my test reader, to my editor who championed this passion project and skillfully guided me to new writing heights, and to all the amazing people I'm truly blessed to have in my life, my sincere gratitude. You all inspire me to be my best self every day!

Contents

1. Get Well

Discovering Natural Remedies

Why did you pick up this book?

Are you stressed and anxious about the state of the world?

Do you have inflammatory or digestive issues?

Can you relate to the 50 million-plus Americans in search of a good night's sleep?[1]

Do you suffer from any of the top health conditions in the United States like major depression, high cholesterol, Crohn's disease, or ulcerative colitis?[2]

Are you one of the six in ten adults who have a chronic disease?[3] Or are you simply curious about how hemp and medicinal plants can fit into your everyday life?

Maybe it's all of the above. And maybe, like me, you believe nature provides the solutions.

You know real is better than fake.

Natural is better than synthetic.

Feeling good is *way* superior to feeling lousy.

When you're stressed out, can't sleep, have a bloated stomach, or just feel run down, everything is harder. When your energy levels are high, your body feels "normal," and your mind is clear, everything is radiant—life is chock full of sunshine. You can take on the world!

Do you want to tackle the stressors of the world with ease? Do you crave better, more natural ways to treat common ailments?

Good news! Nature can support you. It's been doing so for thousands of years.

We are one with the earth—we've evolved together. Plants and humans, we have a long, rewarding, symbiotic relationship.

Many common solutions are already in some of your favorite foods, in the herbs that may already be growing in your garden, and in the luxury bath products you use to unwind at the end of a stressful day. You just haven't learned how to fully harness their medicinal powers. Yet.

Likely, you also picked up this guide because you are more than curious about CBD. Why are you suddenly seeing CBD in every product, in every store? What can it do for you?

Well, thanks to The Hemp Farming Act of 2018, which legalized industrial hemp (with THC concentrations of no more than 0.3 percent), CBD is now in the medicinal plant limelight.

In our lifetime, there's been an awakening, a push for more natural products, artisan craftsmanship, and locally sourced goods. Having lived through the material world of the '80s, it's wildly refreshing for this eco-gal to see the pendulum swing back.

Perhaps, you feel the same?

This global awakening is not only good for our health and happiness, it's good for the health and happiness of the entire planet.

In Slavic mythology, silvan spirits once ruled the forests and meadows. These mountain deities, often known as "wild women," knew all the secrets of nature. They spun hemp, prepared potions, were guardians of the forest, and defenders of nature.

It's time we all once again become wild women (*and men!*).

As a wild person, you can find more natural ways to treat common ailments like stress and anxiety. You will be able to reconnect with nature and start on a better path toward wellness with the aid of medicinal plants.

Simply said—plants help us heal.

Medicinal herbs don't force your body to heal, they don't contradict your natural abilities. What they do is support and encourage your body to find balance and to mend itself. This book offers no cures, but it offers plenty of hope, guidance, knowledge, and encouragement along your quest for natural solutions to common ailments.

My heart is full of joy that you've picked up this guide and have chosen to empower yourself with a deeper understanding of medicinal plants.

We are all part of the earth. The crucial elements for life found in our universe exist within us. We're connected to the cycles of the earth.

If we are off-balance, it simply makes good sense to allow the earth to help restore us!

CBD, HERBS, AND PANDEMICS—OH MY!

I wrote a good portion of this book during the quarantine phase of the COVID-19 pandemic in the United States. This period reinforced not only our need to be more prepared for some major curveballs and the importance of self-reliance, but it also brought to the forefront the great need for better overall health and wellness solutions in our lives.

As we struggled with unanticipated stressors and isolation in our daily routine, discussions about depression, panic attacks, lack of access to fresh produce, and home-schooling challenges quickly became the norm on Facebook. While CBD, hemp, and medicinal gardening aren't an end-all-be-all, I believe they sure could have helped a lot of folks cope better.

Gardening alone is therapeutic. Drinking a warm, delicious, fragrant cup of medicinal tea is comforting, instantly calming the mind, body, and soul. The simple act of dosing a CBD tincture makes you stop, pause, and reflect.

Stress reduction, anxiety alleviation, sleep enhancement, immune-boosting support, mood levelers—all things we searched for in a time of isolation and extreme stress—could have been as close as our kitchen windowsill.

Another issue I became acutely aware of when COVID-19 disrupted our lives is the ridiculous amount of myths and false information that spread faster than the virus. When this happens, people begin accepting myths as facts. Just because you've seen a meme twenty-two times, read multiple articles, or heard a celebrity state a "fact," doesn't make it a truth.

The same lesson applies to cannabis and other medicinal plants. You have to dig deeper!

In *Getting Baked*, I've done a lot of the research for you, interviewed industry experts, and applied my personal expertise with CBD and medicinal gardening. As a writer (with over thirty years' experience in print and digital media), I can say with confidence that nearly all good nonfiction writing stems from quality research on the subject matter.

I also believe all good journeys begin with curiosity, a quest for knowledge, and a passion for the subject matter. You'll totally find my heart poured into these pages. Nature inspires me, and every day I learn something new from our plant world.

I hope you'll find inspiration in these pages and develop a new level of appreciation for our medicinal plant world, too.

This is a starting point for you. If something puzzles you or you find you want to know more about a particular medicinal plant, be sure to ask questions and explore the topic further. There's a wealth of resources available to you. I've listed all my favorites in the last chapter of this guide for your quick reference.

Your personal experience is also a huge part of your myth-busting mission as you dig deeper. Pay attention to the lessons learned from your past experiences and trust your gut instincts.

It's a widely accepted certitude that lavender has a sweet, earthy, desirable flavor. Chefs use it in culinary dishes around the world. Lavender scones are a popular treat you'll find at many coffee houses. You may see it listed as a floral note in a French wine you love. To me, regardless of the preparation method, lavender tastes like perfumed soap (or at least what I imagine perfumed soap to taste like, as I have no desire to take a bite and find out if I'm right!).

That's my personal experience. My truth.

And it's important to integrate this experience into my medicinal garden lifestyle. Despite not appreciating the taste, I love the scent of lavender and extensively use it in topical remedies, bath products, and homemade air fresheners.

I avoid medicinal teas, recipes, and CBD tinctures that contain lavender. I'm fully aware of the health support it offers, but if I don't like the flavor, it's unlikely I'll be able to keep up a health routine that includes ingesting it.

Listen to your body and be mindful of your preferences. If you strongly dislike a medicinal herb, look to a substitute with a similar attribute. Habits begin with mini steps, and the more you enjoy all the benefits of a medicinal plant, including flavor and form, the easier it is to adapt it into your lifestyle.

You may find you're already enjoying plenty of medicinal plants present in this book in your daily diet.

If you love Italian cuisines, chances are you're a big fan of basil and garlic. Perhaps you just don't yet know all the ways you can enjoy these medicinal plants, like using garlic to reduce inflammation and basil to aid with digestives issues.

Some herbs like Holy Basil may be completely new to you. You may have come across mention of Holy Basil reading about Ayurvedic sciences, but chances are you haven't tried growing it in your garden yet, *and you can—it's easy!* (See how in Chapter 4.)

Maybe some medicinal plants, like chamomile, are ones you're already enjoying in your tea rituals, but you never realized their full potential for use as a hair tonic or sleep aid. When paired with CBD oil, chamomile might just give you the restorative, deep sleep you desperately need.

Whatever medicinal plant you choose to begin with in *Getting Baked*, you'll find they are fairly simple to use and/or grow, requiring no extraordinary "green thumb."

What you need is a little know-how.

So, what are we waiting for?

Grab your cup of ashwagandha and peppermint tea (*great for enhancing focus and boosting mental clarity*), and let's get started on our CBD, hemp, and medicinal garden journey!

ARE YOU READY TO GET BAKED?

Medicinal plants are:

- affordable
- accessible
- effective
- empowering

Medicinal plants *are not* a cure.

If you find a medicinal plant or plant extract that cures your ailments—that's freakin' fantastic!

To realistically manage your expectations, though, we'll continue with the tried-and-true philosophy that medicinal plants are not a cure-all.

They also may have side effects or interact with over-the-counter (OTC) drugs or prescriptions. They may interfere with medicines or supplements you're already taking. The information in this guide is not medical advice, nor a substitute for your doctor's care.

What we are exploring is a lifestyle choice, which may potentially enhance your efforts to bring new relief and support where it is much needed.

Always consult your doctor, pharmacist, nutritionist, and other health practitioners before adding medicinal plants to your health routines. It's just smart to keep everyone who is concerned with your personal health needs in the loop.

Medicinal plants should be treated as companions. They are partners in your health and wellness journey on the path toward better health, one awesome facet of a holistic approach.

We all know that to keep a car running, all parts of the vehicle must be in good repair and work in harmony. The same is true with our bodies. It's just as important to address your feelings and moods as it is to repair your digestive system.

For example: For many years, I struggled not only to get to sleep, but to stay asleep.

You don't need to read a study to understand the importance of quality sleep—we all know this from personal experience. Sleep is a significant component of your overall health and well-being. When you sleep well, you feel better, think more clearly, and your entire body functions at a higher level.

A few years ago, my husband and I decided to purchase a new bed in hopes of getting better rest. It helped a bit. I added supportive pillows to keep my body aligned correctly for optimum sleep. It certainly added some comfort each night.

I tried dozens of techniques, from meditation to ambient noise machines. Each added a modicum of aid in my efforts. In addition, I adjusted my diet to restrict caffeine to morning consumption only, and I exercised during the day to ensure my lifestyle wasn't too sedentary.

All these steps aided my efforts to achieve a good night's rest each night, but none completely solved my insomnia.

That's when I turned to herbs and later to full-spectrum CBD. By using them in combination together and with the above changes in my lifestyle, I've finally achieved my goal—a lovely night's rest each night with a deep, restorative sleep.

There's an Irish proverb I grew up hearing: *A good laugh and a long sleep are the best cures.*

I never fully understood this proverb until I began to have sleep problems and then eventually found solutions. My ancestors sure were onto something! When you are well rested, every other element of your life, from your emotional to spiritual well-being, is easier to address, both the good and the bad aspects.

The thing about sleep (*or any ailment*) is there's not a one-step solution for most people. It's important to take a holistic approach. In my personal example, the ultimate key to my fully having restorative sleep is full-spectrum CBD and medicinal herbs used in combination with addressing my environmental, dietary, and cognitive needs.

CBD and medicinal herbs are no-nonsense, easily accessible solutions that aid my overall health objectives and bring them to a tangible, rewarding solution. Best of all, the steps I've taken and all the medicinal plants I use are super easy to incorporate into my lifestyle.

This easy-breezy philosophy is what I hope you'll take to heart. *Getting Baked* is designed to be a guide for the everyday herbalist, no prior experience required. You'll find easily recognizable plants and plant compounds you may already be familiar with and step-by-step instructions to follow.

Sure, I love the idea of creating a wizard-like potion lab in my garden and home (*and I do grow some exotics just for fun*), but why would we not take advantage of what already surrounds us? Why mess with Motherwort (*a plant most of us are not familiar with*) for headache pain when Peppermint (*a plant we're likely to be awfully familiar with*) is already available to us?

There's also a level of fear involved with plants and ingredients we're not familiar with. For good reason, we should approach them with caution and learn the basics in order to gain the confidence to continue forward.

You can take your medicinal garden journey as far as you wish to go. Just like any path of learning, though, it's best to begin with building blocks we're familiar with in the same way we learn the alphabet before we learn to read. Take your journey one step at a time. Listen to your body and take a holistic approach toward finding your perfect balance.

For example: If sleep is your primary health concern, there are many easy steps you can take.

1. **Identify** the medicinal plants in *Getting Baked* that may be of aid in enhancing your sleep efforts, like full-spectrum CBD, lavender, ashwagandha, and chamomile. (*I've included plenty of handy charts throughout the guide for your reference.*)

2. **Check in** with your doctor, pharmacist, and other health practitioners to discuss underlying causes for your ailments. Also discuss potential drug interactions with CBD or the medicinal plants you're planning to use as part of your treatment. Always be your own advocate!

3. **Introduce** each medicinal plant companion to your path one at a time to assess its effectiveness.

4. **Grow** and process the plants that work best for you. Find the ideal ways to incorporate them into your daily routine in *Getting Baked*. I've included everything from topicals to edibles to bath and beauty product suggestions for you to try.

5. **Take inventory** of your environment to see if you might need adjustments like light-blocking curtains for your bedroom.

6. **Be mindful** of your diet and eliminate habits like late-night snacking that might be interfering with your sleep cycle.

7. **Tune in** to your emotions and address your stress levels with mindful activities like yoga or meditation.

8. **Have an intuitive conversation** with your body and assess if your lifestyle is too sedentary. Adding more movement to your day may be a piece of the puzzle you need to add in to complete your wellness solution.

These steps may sound like a lot, but they're absolutely not! You can quickly lay out a plan for yourself for every health and wellness need you have.

Plenty of the commonsense stuff we already know:

· Most whole foods are better than processed foods
· Chemicals are generally not healthy for our bodies.
· Regular exercise is good for us.

You don't need a complex formula to realize that if you burn more calories than you consume, you typically lose weight and often rest better. We just need to make our health and wellness a priority (and obviously you're already starting to since you picked up this guide, so bravo!).

The cooking, gardening, dosing, and crafting ideas highlighted in *Getting Baked* are all part of the holistic approach you not only need, but deep down inside, you crave. In the end, every single step is worth the effort when the end result is better health!

I always chuckle when I hear the term *alternative health*. Good health should be the target, not an alternative.

Natural remedies are not alternatives, they are part of nature, existing way before any synthetic solution. When we take care of ourselves and seek natural solutions, we opt out of the synthetic drug cycle that's often dragging us down with an endless array of harmful side effects.

This is not to say that modern science and modern drug therapies don't serve a role in improving our health and wellness. But they are often one of many solutions available, including "alternative" health aids like medicinal plants.

Nature provides many solutions. It's just plain smart to work in harmony with our natural environment.

After all, nature always finds a way. Now it's time for you to find your natural path!

 FRESH-BAKED TIP: The journal pages and lists included in *Getting Baked* are available for free download at: http://www.ruralmom.com/getting-baked

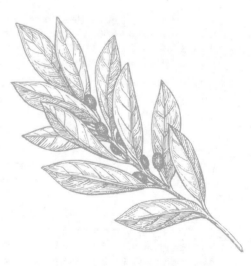

2. Get Baked

Understanding Hemp, CBD, and the Cannabis Culture

Energizing, alluring, soothing, uplifting, euphoric—enticing words that could describe a famous work of art or an expensive perfume. They're also terms used to describe the characteristics of cannabis.

Touted in ancient times as an "elixir of life," cannabis can be found throughout literature, mythology, archaeology, agriculture, and scientific studies.

Archeology findings show Vikings cultivated hemp around 650 AD.[4] Excavation work in Turkey revealed samples of hemp-woven fabric, dating back 9,000 years.[5] Greek historian Herodotus recorded inhaling vapors of hemp-seed smoke in fifth century BC[6]

Yet, cannabis is the most misunderstood flowering plant in history. Debates about marijuana and industrial hemp continue today as the agricultural, medical, scientific, and wellness communities continue to explore the many facets of this fascinating herb.

HOW CANNABIS SAVVY ARE YOU?

Can you tell fact from fiction? How well do you know your facts about CBD and hemp?

Take this epic quiz to test your knowledge!

Below are ten statements. Determine whether you think the statement is true or if it is a myth. When you're finished, read the answers in the next section to see how well you did.

1	Smoking or ingesting CBD will get you high.	TRUTH	MYTH
2	Cannabis is the solution for curing cancer, eliminating global warming, and solving world peace.	TRUTH	MYTH
3	Hemp, CBD, and marijuana are all the same.	TRUTH	MYTH
4	CBD has been scientifically proven to help with some health conditions.	TRUTH	MYTH
5	There is THC in hempseed oil.	TRUTH	MYTH
6	Hempseed oil can be used as fuel for automobiles.	TRUTH	MYTH
7	The Declaration of Independence is written on hemp paper.	TRUTH	MYTH
8	Levi's, Patagonia, and TOMS use hemp fabrics in their fashions.	TRUTH	MYTH
9	Taking CBD will cause you to test positive on a drug test.	TRUTH	MYTH
10	All CBD is created equally.	TRUTH	MYTH

SCORING: Give yourself one point for each correct answer. Tally up the points to obtain your total score.

1–3 points: You may be new to the cannabis culture, but by the end of this book, you'll be delighting your friends with all kinds of fun facts.

4–6 points: A cannabis lover at heart, you have a good foundation of knowledge. Continue reading this chapter to fill in the blanks.

7–10 points: You're a cannabis quiz star. You sure know your facts and will love discovering new ways to incorporate CBD and hemp into your lifestyle. Read on!

Statement 1: MYTH—CBD does not have a psychoactive effect.

Tetrahydrocannabinol, otherwise known as THC, is the compound in cannabis that is psychotropic. CBD stands for cannabidiol, one of the many other compounds found in the cannabis plant.

In accordance with current regulations in the United States, legal CBD products must be extracted from industrial hemp plants containing levels of less than .3 percent THC. Because of this, legal CBD products are nonintoxicating.

For people with concerns about any level of THC in a CBD product, there are CBD products available that contain zero THC. We'll be discussing this in more depth later in this chapter.

Statement 2: MYTH—It would be lovely if cannabis could cure all the world's problems, but alas, it is not a cure-all.

Cannabis does, however, have some amazing properties and applications. Medical professionals and scientists are studying how cannabis can help with many diseases, including various types of cancer. It takes fewer resources to create plastics, fabrics, paper, and other products from hemp, which could reduce our eco-footprint.

As for world peace, well, no one plant can bring that about. It will take more than a cannabis culture village to succeed!

Statement 3: TRUTH (also give yourself credit if you answered MYTH)—The truth is hemp and marijuana are derived from the same plant, genus *Cannabis* in the family *Cannabaceae*.

The most recognizable difference between marijuana and hemp is the level of THC within the plant. Marijuana has high levels of THC (over .3 percent). Industrial hemp (often referred to as "hemp," and for all practical purposes what I am referring to when I use the term "hemp" throughout this guide) is currently defined as a cannabis plant containing less than .3 percent THC.

CBD is a compound found in the cannabis plant. So technically, it's not the same as hemp and marijuana—it is derived from hemp and marijuana plants. (This is why you get to give yourself credit if you answered MYTH.)

Statement 4: TRUTH—There have been many scientific studies conducted that have shown that CBD can help with some health conditions, and there are numerous studies currently in progress. I'll be referencing many of these studies throughout the guide, and you'll find additional helpful resources in the last chapter of this guide in case you'd like to investigate further.

Earlier studies on CBD's effectiveness in treating epilepsy have led to the Food and Drug Administration (FDA) approval of the prescription drug Epidiolex.[7] This drug contains a purified form of CBD that is used to treat seizure disorders.

Statement 5: MYTH—Hempseed oil is not a source of THC.

It is possible that a minute trace of THC or any of the other multitude of cannabis compounds could be found in hempseed oil.

The trace, however, is miniscule, like the way poppy seeds on your bagel contain trace elements of opiates.[8] No matter how many bagels you scarf down with your morning coffee, you won't get high. However, you may have a really big tummy ache.

Statement 6: TRUTH—Hemp can be used to produce more than 25,000 products,[9] including fuel for diesel automobiles. Diesel engines are designed to run on organic fuels like hempseed oil.

Statement 7: MYTH—The Declaration of Independence is not written on hemp paper.

This common myth is perpetuated by the fact that popular patriots like Thomas Jefferson and George Washington grew hemp at their estates. While it's possible that drafts of the declaration were written on paper derived from hemp, according to the National Archives, the Declaration of Independence is written on parchment paper,[10] typically produced at the time from treated animal skin.

Statement 8: TRUTH—Levi's, Patagonia, and TOMS do use hemp fabrics in their fashions.

Hemp fiber is some of the strongest, most absorbent, elastic, and durable of the natural fibers available. It's been used for centuries to create clothing and other textiles. The Levi's Wellthread collection uses cottonized hemp,[11] Patagonia is well known for using hemp fibers in their clothing collections,[12] and TOMS Earthwise products contain eco-friendly fibers including hemp.[13]

Statement 9: TRUTH—Some forms of CBD may cause you to test positive on a drug test.[14]

Full-spectrum CBD and CBD distillate products do contain trace amounts of THC. Broad-spectrum and CBD isolate products are THC-free. (More information on the differences between these product formats can be found later in this chapter.)

You should take this into consideration when determining which CBD product will be the best fit for you. If you have concerns about testing THC positive on a drug test, seek out products with zero THC.

Statement 10: MYTH—CBD is a natural compound found in the cannabis plant, but CBD products are not all created equally.

CBD products are created through various means, including synthetic production. In its natural form, various distillation methods also exist to extract the CBD compound from cannabis. They each deliver a different variation of the product. (We'll be covering these more in-depth later in this chapter.)

AN HERB BY ANY OTHER NAME

How did you do on the quiz? Did you already know all of hemp's superpowers? Or, like me, were you (initially) surprised by some of the cannabis myths and truths?

Books, archives, documentaries, websites, scientific studies, and oodles of additional resources are dedicated to unraveling all the myths and mysteries of this awe-inducing herb. Hemp's numerous applications are nearly as complex as the plant itself.

In this book, we are focused on integrating industrial hemp products and cannabidiol (CBD) into your current regimes and lifestyle. When you form a new habit, it's so much easier if it matches up with habits you already have, isn't it?

One thing that may not be so straightforward and easy to understand, though, is CBD. It's a new frontier we're exploring, so it's especially important to have a clear understanding of all the ABC's and 123's of CBD.

You've probably noticed by now that CBD is everywhere! Increasing your understanding of cannabidiol may be what prompted you to pick up this book.

Does CBD really do anything? How helpful is it? What product should you choose? From CBD gummies to pillows and exercise gear—navigating this fascinating compound molecule can be overwhelming. It doesn't need to be.

The three keys you need to help you find your way through the cannabidiol maze are:

1. Learning what CBD is
2. Understanding how it works
3. Discovering how to select the best CBD product(s) for you

Let's get started and unlock all the mysteries of CBD.

We're going to dip into the science of CBD briefly because it's both fascinating and important to understand. If the mere mention of science makes you yawn or brings up dreaded memories of icky high school lab moments, I totally get that. Throughout my early school years, science classes mainly boggled my mind.

Then I found that one teacher—you know, the wonderful one who suddenly explains things in a way that makes everything clearer—and suddenly science was fun and made sense. I'm going to try to be that teacher as we take a peek at the process, and I promise, there will be no test afterward, so take all the time you need to digest the info.

A LITTLE COMPOUND CALLED CBD

CBD is a molecule found in cannabis plants.

It's one of many cannabinoids in cannabis plants, but it's not present, naturally, in abundance.

The cannabis plant family includes hemp and marijuana. Most consumer CBD products are extracted from hemp plants, not marijuana plants.

Initially, CBD is part of a cannabidiolic acid known as CBDa. Heating a hemp flower, a process called decarboxylation, releases CBD from CBDa. There are also other methods of harvesting CBD, but this is a common one.

We could delve deeper into the process, but in a nutshell: An extraction procedure pulls CBD oil from the flowers, stalks, and/or seeds of the hemp plant. CBD oil extractions are then typically mixed with base oils like coconut oil, MCT oil, or hempseed oil. These base oils are called "carriers" that help dilute the CBD, making it easier for your body to absorb it.

Usually ingested or used topically, CBD oil is often used by people to reduce inflammation, improve mood, or enhance sleep. Studies have shown CBD to have potential benefits for people who have arthritis, epilepsy, chronic pain, and PTSD.[15]

Anecdotally throughout history, CBD has been shown to help with acne, migraines, depression, anxiety, insomnia, and inflammation.

CBD works in conjunction with the body's endocannabinoid system. This system was defined by scientists in the early 1990s. Its main purpose is believed to be the regulation of bodily functions to maintain equilibrium (homeostasis) in the body. The endocannabinoid system is like having a team of crossing guards in your body. The crossing guards (receptors) interpret traffic lights (signals) as they act and react to vehicles on the road (internal and external stimuli). In other words, the receptors in your body work together with molecules called endocannabinoids that signal the receptors to make sure your body stays in balance as it meets with various changes to your internal and external environment.

This system, just like a school crossing guard, helps create harmony and compliance at the "crosswalk."

There are two main receptors (crossing guards) in the endocannabinoid system: CB1 and CB2.

RECEPTOR	INTERACTS WITH
CB1	bone marrow, brain, gastrointestinal tract, immune system, liver, lungs, muscles, pancreas, vascular system
CB2	bone marrow, bones, immune system, liver, pancreas, spleen, skin

Our body naturally produces endocannabinoid molecules in response to things like hunger, stress, exercise, and pain. These endocannabinoids help us in various ways, such as alleviating pain or stimulating our appetite. They bind to the CB1 and CB2 receptors to signal what our bodies need.

Scientists learned that CBD and THC, natural cannabinoids found in cannabis, mimic the endocannabinoids we naturally produce.[16] Because of this, molecules like CBD or THC can disrupt our endocannabinoid system and create new responses.

For example, THC switches off our endocannabinoid system. This produces the "high" we associate with marijuana.

 FRESH-BAKED TIP: CBD also interacts with our endovanilloid system,[17] which is the system in our body that triggers us to experience a hot effect from hot peppers or a cooling effect from herbs like peppermint.

CBD interacts with many of the receptors in our bodies. It prevents our own compounds from binding to the receptors.[18] The effects we feel from this may vary by person. Just as our DNA is unique to us, so are the actions and reactions of receptors in our endocannabinoid system.

Therefore, some people experience a mood-lifting experience or pain relief when using CBD, and others do not. Our own endocannabinoids are designed to be precise for our own body. The effects of cannabinoids like CBD are imprecise.

However, the more we learn about CBD and other cannabinoids, the more potential it appears to have as a treatment option for many common illnesses.

Other plants, including one we are awfully familiar with—cacao (used to produce chocolate)— also contain compounds that interact with our endocannabinoid system.

Cacao contains anandamide, a lipid that interacts with cannabinoid receptors in a way that boosts our mood.[19] This is why some people experience a happy feeling after consuming a chocolate bar or a cup of hot cocoa. It's not all about just the joy the delicious taste brings us!

IS CBD FOR ME?

With CBD, you must be your own health advocate. There is no all-encompassing solution or path.

Janson Hoambrecker, cannabis expert and CEO of Hempton Farms (hemptonfarms.com), a CBD seed-to-table producer, suggests listening to your body first and foremost. "The big thing is, we don't know what we don't know," says Hoambrecker. "We know this plant has amazing characteristics, but it's not a one size fits all cure."

Because of prior strict laws on growing cannabis in the United States, a lot of the information we have on the effects of CBD is anecdotal. We'll continue to see more and more research as the laws continue to change.

By 2020, eleven states have legalized marijuana for recreational use, thirty-three states have legalized marijuana for medical use, and forty-eight have allowed OTC sales of CBD products. Yet, for our north neighbors in Canada, CBD is available by prescription only.

Due to COVID-19, which raised awareness of complications for people with lung issues, and a rising number of deaths in 2019 attributed to inferior vape cartridges from illicit manufacturers (known in the cannabis culture as "Vapegate"), CBD in an inhalable format is in less demand. The demand for CBD oral and edible products still seems to be on the upswing, though, as more people discover the potential benefits.

"Education is king," says Hoambrecker. "The more Americans get educated on what the power of CBD can do, the more we can get past the stigmas."

Ultimately, to decide if CBD is right for you, listen to your body, read the right materials (like *Getting Baked!*), and work with your doctor(s).

It's also important to keep in mind that CBD by itself may not be the key to alleviating your ailments. You may find that daily use of CBD, lavender, and turmeric is your key to reducing inflammation and stress. Or you may need to alter your diet along with taking CBD.

If you're not working in harmony with your body, you're defeating your intentions. If you're using CBD to reduce inflammation in your body but consuming large quantities of sugar-filled soft drinks or processed meat each week (two foods known to cause inflammation[20]), you're setting yourself up to fail. As Plato wrote in *Charmides*, "The part can never be well unless the whole is well."[21]

Much like coffee, CBD comes from a plant, can be consumed daily, and will have varied effects depending upon the user.

Studies show that up to 1500 milligrams (mg) of CBD is well tolerated by the body.[22] The World Health Organization (WHO) finds that "no public health problems have been associated with CBD use."[23]

Currently, what we know is CBD is a natural plant ingredient with therapeutic potential. If you've decided CBD is for you, keep reading because now that you understand what it is and how it works, the next step is to learn how to select the best product for you.

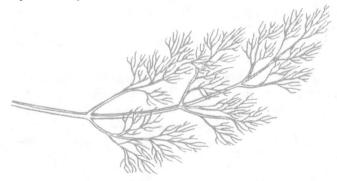

DID SOMEONE SAY GUMMY BEARS?

New products with CBD as an ingredient are hitting store shelves daily. While your options seem endless, there are ultimately three main forms for CBD available: oral, topical, and inhalable.

- **Oral forms of CBD** include strips, oils, tinctures, and edibles (like gummies, chocolates, and coffee).
- **Topical forms of CBD** include oils, creams, salves, and lip balms.
- **Inhalable forms of CBD** include vapes, flowers, and concentrates (like waxes and shatters).

Each of these product forms delivers CBD to your endocannabinoid system at different speeds. Inhalation benefits are immediate but have a shorter duration of effect. Oral consumption takes longer but the effects also last longer. Topicals generally offer immediate relief for a moderate duration (one to three hours).

Each person may react differently to each form. The forms can be combined to create your own custom regimen. To determine which product will work best for you, first ask "What am I treating?"

 FRESH-BAKED TIP: According the WHO, "CBD is generally well tolerated with a good safety profile."[24] However, there may be side effects like drowsiness,[25] dry mouth,[26] or lowered blood pressure,[27] with use.

Dehydration is a side effect I regularly have after ingesting CBD, so I always ensure I chase each dose with a full glass of water and stay well hydrated throughout the day. As I also use CBD as a sleep aid. In the morning, water is the first thing I reach for to replenish my body.

The FDA Consumer Update outlines safety concerns related to CBD products including potential liver injury, interactions with other drugs, and drowsiness.[28] It also stresses that there is much yet to learn about CBD and its effects, including any effect it may have on fetuses and newborns (for pregnant or breastfeeding women). You can access the most current information regarding CBD and other consumer products at fda.gov/consumers.

Some people may also have cannabis allergies. If you are taking prescription medications, there are potential interactions. Always err on the safe side and consult your doctor and pharmacist prior to use.

To date, CBD is not considered an addictive substance. If you decide to try CBD, you should have no symptoms of withdrawal if you miss a dose or stop taking it. Like any supplement, though, if you are taking CBD for a specific condition like anxiety and you decide to stop taking it, you may have a return of the symptoms you helped alleviate.

The form of CBD is one piece of the puzzle. Other important pieces to understand are types of CBD available, dosage, ratios, and terpenes.

ONE PILL HAS A LITTLE, ONE PILL HAS NONE

There are four common types of CBD products currently manufactured:

1. CBD isolate
2. CBD distillate
3. Full-Spectrum CBD
4. Broad-Spectrum CBD

One of the most important characteristics of CBD isolate is that it's THC-free.

In simple terms, to create a CBD isolate, the CBD compound is isolated and removed from the hemp plant. This typically results in a nearly 100 percent pure CBD powder. Everything else is filtered out. There are no other cannabinoids (like THC), plant oils, terpenes (which will be explained later in this chapter), or other plant matter present.

For people who are THC sensitive or wish to avoid consuming THC or other cannabis cannabinoids or plant matter, CBD isolate is a good choice to consider. CBD isolate is also flavorless. This can be a bonus for people who do not enjoy the earthy plant flavors commonly associated with cannabis.

A CBD distillate, unlike isolate, is not a pure form of CBD. It may contain other cannabinoids (including THC), terpenes, and cannabis plant materials. CBD distillates often contain higher levels of THC, potentially exceeding the .3 percent allowable by federal law, as it's typically sourced from marijuana, not hemp plants.

In contrast, full-spectrum CBD has a high concentration of CBD, and also includes a full array of other cannabinoids (including THC), terpenes, and plant matter *but* maintains the THC level under the .3 percent allowable. Full-spectrum products that include all the natural cannabinoids, terpenes, and other assets like vitamins and minerals available from the hemp plant are often touted as having an "entourage effect." Think of the entourage effect just like the word "entourage" implies.

For example: By yourself you can have fun participating in an activity like walking. When a group of your best friends (aka your *entourage*) join you, you are affected, generally in a positive way. Your walk will be more enjoyable as you chat and pass time with people who lift you up and add a new level of fun to your journey.

Cannabis compounds work the same way. CBD is pretty awesome on its own, but add all its plant friends (other cannabinoids, essential oils, terpenes, and so on) to the mix, and they boost each other in positive ways.

If you are THC sensitive, however, a full-spectrum product may have mild sedative effects. This is great if sleep is your objective, but not so great if you are using CBD during the daytime in hopes of reducing inflammation in your body.

If you have concerns that THC is present in full-spectrum products, to put it in perspective: we've learned by law that a full-spectrum product derived from industrial hemp must contain less than .3 percent THC. Marijuana plants typically contain over 20 percent THC. In contrast, .3 percent is a miniscule amount.

Advocates in the industrial hemp industry are trying to change the laws to allow potentially 1 percent THC in industrial hemp to be the new farming standard. The driving factor behind this is the harsh penalization for farmers who grow industrial hemp that may exceed the arbitrary .3 standard. In farming, exceeding that limit is easier to do than one might think. The chemistry of a hemp plant changes by genetics, climate, soil factors, and other environmental influences just like any other plant.

You'll find the same to be true when you tend to your medicinal garden. Some plants will thrive and meet record highs for growth, others will wilt and you'll have to figure out what variable is causing it to have a different growth pattern.

For a farmer who may have a hemp crop that tests at .4 THC due to optimum growing conditions or an organic fertilizer that affected the plant's growth in a positive way, they are at risk of having their entire crop destroyed, along with facing potential criminal charges. (You can learn more about this issue at agriculturalhempsolutions.com.)

Even if a 1 percent allowance is approved, marijuana plants will still be twenty times more potent than industrial hemp plants.

The 1 percent allowable in the field may not necessarily mean there will be a 1 percent trace of THC in full-spectrum CBD products, either. Depending upon the method used, the extraction process will reduce the THC level prior to producing the end product for packaging.

Regardless, the likelihood that you will ever get "high" from a legally produced CBD product is not a reasonable deduction. The exorbitant cost of attempting to use full-spectrum CBD to ever catch even a small buzz is prohibitive, especially when a less-expensive viable alternative like marijuana exists.

If you are THC sensitive, or you need high doses of CBD and are concerned that will increase your THC consumption, broad-spectrum CBD is a great option to consider. Broad-spectrum CBD has a high concentration of CBD and contains an array of cannabinoids, terpenes, and hemp plant matter. However, THC is removed from broad-spectrum products.

For people who are in search of the "entourage effect," but don't wish to use a product with THC, broad-spectrum is also a good choice.

FULL-SPECTRUM CBD	BROAD-SPECTRUM CBD	CBD ISOLATE	CBD DISTILLATE
CBD, additional naturally occurring cannabinoids, terpenes, flavonoids, essential oils, plant matter.	CBD, additional naturally occurring cannabinoids, terpenes, flavonoids, essential oils, plant matter.	CBD, no other cannabis plant material.	CBD, some additional naturally occurring cannabinoids, terpenes, and plant matter.
THC < .3 %	**No THC**	**No THC**	**THC may be > .3 %**

 FRESH-BAKED TIP: There are plenty of cannabinoids in cannabis. Estimates range upward of 100 in total.

THC and CBD are the two most common cannabinoids found and generally, the most plentiful. Most other cannabinoids are found in smaller or minute levels. Some of the more recognizable minor cannabinoids you may see highlighted or discussed are:

- **CBC**—Cannabichromene. A nonintoxicating cannabinoid that interacts with endocannabinoid system receptors, primarily for pain perception. CBC is being studied for its potential in treating cancer patients.
- **CBG**—Cannabigerol. Currently the subject of several studies for potential application for things like glaucoma treatment, inflammatory bowel disease treatment, and appetite stimulation.
- **CBN**—Cannabinol. This cannabinoid is found to increase as a cannabis plant ages. It's being studied for its potential as an antibacterial agent.

WHAT SHOULD MY CBD DOSAGE BE?

Remember the fairy tale of Goldilocks and how she had to find the porridge that was "just right"?

For some people, like me, an overdose of CBD will make them extremely tired. If I pump my body full of CBD, I'm going to sleep really, really well. It's the perfect porridge if my objective is sleep, but completely wrong if I'm just seeking some inflammation relief.

Even if I want to use CBD for sleep, which I often do, I still don't want to overload my body with it. I must find the optimal dose that helps me achieve the perfect night of rest I crave.

According the Centers for Disease Control and Prevention (CDC), more research is needed to determine the ideal dosage amount of CBD per person.[29] Factors like the condition you're treating and your personal body chemistry may affect the dose you need. A great place to begin deciding what dose is right for you is to consult your doctor, pharmacist, or other health professionals you're working with.

If you have chronic pain, it's likely you may need a higher dose than someone seeking support for anxiety or hoping to enhance their quality of sleep. Every expert I've interacted with, interviewed, or spoken with casually over the past few years who is involved in the cannabis industry has had the same exact advice: Start low and go slow.

Begin your CBD journey with a low dose of CBD and slowly increase it if necessary. This pattern continues until you find what optimally works for you.

After trial and error, I personally found that 25 mg of full-spectrum CBD taken daily in the morning works well with my overall mood enhancement and helps alleviate carpal tunnel symptoms. Another 10 to 25 mg taken in the late evening helps me sleep soundly through the night.

Garo Keresteci, founding partner of FUSE Create and owner of Canna-Commerce.com, says the biggest challenge he sees in the cannabis industry is dosage. "What amount works? It's very tough to know what is optimum or not," says Keresteci. "We know what an aspirin does, but what is the appropriate dosage of CBD? It's a complicated area with so many verticals to consider. Clearly, we have a need for more data."

The industry will continue to evolve, and we are likely to see a better set of standards for dosage soon. Keresteci suggests consulting your health care practitioners for dosage advice and educating yourself by keeping up with current research.

You can stay up to date with regulations and research by utilizing the resource guide in Chapter 10 of *Getting Baked*.

Also be mindful that dosage should be clearly stated on a package.

For example: A package of CBD gummies may state that the overall content of the package contains 150 mg of CBD and each piece (dose) contains 10 mg. That way you know that each gummy you consume should be delivering 10 mg of CBD. Or that if you opt to consume the entire package, you will consume a total of 150 mg of CBD.

As a liquid product, CBD oil will list dosage by milliliter. A typical bottle will have 15 milliliters (ml), and the bottle dropper will generally dose 1 ml servings. Therefore, if a 15 ml bottle contains 600 mg of CBD, then each dropperful of 1 ml will contain a 40 mg dose of CBD. Half a dropperful (.5 ml) will have a dose of 20 mg of CBD.

Here's a handy chart for your reference for CBD oil to help you understand how many milligrams of CBD are in each 1 ml dropperful.

MILLIGRAMS OF CBD PER 1 ML DROPPERFUL			
CBD mg per bottle	15 ml bottle	30 ml bottle	60 ml bottle
100 mg	6.67 mg	3.34 mg	1.67 mg
150 mg	10 mg	5 mg	2.5 mg
250 mg	16.67 mg	8.34 mg	4.17 mg
350 mg	23.34 mg	11.67 mg	5.84 mg

MILLIGRAMS OF CBD PER 1 ML DROPPERFUL (cont.)			
450 mg	30 mg	15 mg	7.5 mg
500 mg	33.34 mg	16.67 mg	8.34 mg
550 mg	36.67 mg	18.34 mg	9.17 mg
750 mg	50 mg	25 mg	12.5 mg
1000 mg	66.67 mg	33.34 mg	16.67 mg
1500 mg	100 mg	50 mg	25 mg
3000 mg	200 mg	100 mg	50 mg

An important aspect of dosing is not only to understand how much you're consuming but to also be consistent with your dose. Like with any supplement, taking it regularly keeps the product in your system, doing the work you expect it to do and generally building effectiveness over time.

Taking CBD for a day and expecting miracles is not realistic. You may, indeed, experience immediate relief or a great night's sleep on the very first day. The key, though, is to incorporate it into your lifestyle over at least a three- to four-week period to be able to have a clear understanding of how well the supplement is working for you.

Again, low and slow. Start with a small dose, take it daily for several weeks to gauge the effectiveness. Then increase your dosage slowly if you need more.

WHAT'S THE RIGHT CBD RATIO?

The ratio of CBD in the product is referring to the ratio of CBD to THC.

The higher the CBD level is to THC, the more benefits you will receive from CBD and the less "high" you may feel from the THC present in the product. For example: an 18:1 (CBD/THC) ratio means the CBD is much higher than the THC levels. You should expect to have pain or stress relief with no "high" at all.

A 1:1 (CBD/THC) ratio means the CBD and THC are present in equal proportions. Depending upon the dose, there may be some mild effects, such as a "high" feeling from the THC.

A 1:2 (CBD/THC) ratio is often a dose that you will see prescribed for chronic pain or various illnesses. This is a typical ratio for marijuana.

Ratio is more of a concern to those living in states where medical or recreational marijuana is legal. In states where marijuana is not legal, the ratio of THC should always be much lower than its CBD counterpart as, by current law, industrial hemp must contain less than .3 percent THC.

WHAT IN THE HECK ARE TERPENES AND WHY SHOULD I CARE?

Terpenes are organic compounds that give plants, flowers, and herbs their unique aromas, colors, and flavors. Plants use them to attract pollinators and repel predators. They're also found in hemp plants. Factors that affect the terpene level in a plant include soil and environment.

Terpenes, when paired with cannabinoids like CBD, create what we referred to previously as an "entourage effect." They work in harmony to enhance natural healing properties. When present, terpenes play a role in the taste and effects of a CBD product.

Most of what we know about cannabis terpenes is anecdotal. This will likely change as soon as researchers continue to delve into the study of cannabis terpenes. Some of the common terpenes you will find in cannabis are:

TERPENE	COMMONLY ASSOCIATED ATTRIBUTES
LIMONENE	Citrus aroma. Used to aid with digestion and reducing stress.
MYRCENE	Musky aroma. Used as an anti-inflammatory and sedative.

TERPENE	COMMONLY ASSOCIATED ATTRIBUTES (cont.)
NEROLIDOL	Floral, woody aroma. Used for anxiety and as a sedative.
ALPHA-PINENE + BETA-PINENE	Pine tree aroma. Used as an anti-inflammatory and to improve airflow in respiratory system.
LINALOOL	Floral, spicy aroma. Used for its calming effects, often for relaxing or as a sedative.
HUMULENE	Woody, earthy, spicy aroma. Used for pain relief and as an anti-inflammatory.
TERPINEOL	Floral, citrusy aroma. Used as an antioxidant.

Just like CBD, each terpene may have a different effect for each person.

For example: The herb lavender contains linalool. Some people find this terpene to induce a feeling of calmness. Others turn their nose up at the scent and do not experience any sense of relaxation.

Terpenes are a significant ingredient in essential oils. They are what gives lavender its lovely, relaxing scent and basil its delightful, peppery taste.

Limonene is found in spearmint, celeriac, dill, and basil. Myrcene in rosemary, oregano, and cardamom. Peppers, basil, and tarragon all have the terpene Nerolidol. All the popular terpenes found in hemp are also found in many herb and spices.

Black pepper, cinnamon, and cannabis all contain a terpene called beta-caryophyllene (BCP). This terpene is strongly associated with peppery aromas and tastes. Scientists discovered BCP acts like a dietary cannabinoid, binding to the CB2 receptor, where it has an anti-inflammatory effect.[30]

As we continue to connect the dots, it's clear to see why CBD and medicinal herbs have a wonderful natural love connection.

How to Choose the Best CBD Options for You

There's a southernism that goes "Just 'cuz a chicken has wings, don't mean it can fly." The same applies to CBD products. No matter how colorful, quirky, or farm fresh the label looks, its appearance may be deceiving.

There are six attributes you should take into consideration when you look at a CBD product label:

1. Appearance
2. Ingredients
3. Effects
4. Origin
5. Lab Tests
6. Price

Whenever I have a friend who tells me CBD isn't working for them, nearly every time we discover that they're not seeing any results because they are using an inferior product.

When you're considering using CBD, you must do your homework. You need to take the time to ensure the product you're purchasing is of high quality and designed to treat the ailments you are seeking support for.

APPEARANCE—WHY AM I SO ATTRACTED TO THIS CBD PRODUCT?

Appearance is an important factor to consider when looking at a CBD product. Brands often create eye-catching labels to attract your attention. Personally, I love a sleek package design as they appeal to my minimalist nature. But I also want to quickly find all the information I need and not have to work through a puzzle of colors, patterns, or slogans.

A pioneer in the Illinois hemp farming industry and cofounder of Half Day CBD, Kameron Norwood has some great insights on what consumers should be looking for in CBD product labeling. Half Day CBD (www.halfdaycbd.com) is a U.S.-based company that works directly with Illinois farmers, local processors, and manufacturers to create their products in a commercial kitchen in Chicago.

After admiring Half Day CBD's clean yet colorful packaging (and their coffee-flavored CBD gummies), I had the chance to dig deeper and chat with Norwood about consumer education. As he's worked in all facets of the industry, he has a good handle on the pitfalls both manufacturers and consumers face.

Norwood suggests consumers look past the glitz of the label, but do pay attention to the style. "Ask 'What brand speaks to me?'" says Norwood. "Some brands are more medical. Others are more work-focused, fun, or serene. Some are just gimmicky, so beware."

Norwood suggests beginning with the brands that speak to you first and to do your due diligence to investigate further. Does the brand address the area of concern you need support with? How will it aid you?

"Clarity is an important feature to look for. Contact information should be easy to find. Third-party reviews and lab tests should be present," says Norwood. "And ingredients should be easily identifiable and understood."

INGREDIENTS—WHAT ON EARTH IS IN THIS CBD PRODUCT?

First and foremost, CBD should be listed as an ingredient on the package. You should be able to clearly understand how many milligrams of CBD are in each serving and in the entire package.

You might be thinking "Duh, of course CBD should be in the CBD product." You're right, but unfortunately, due to a lack of regulations, yet-to-be-clearly-defined standards, and the boom of the CBD industry, you will find there are plenty of companies making false claims.

One of these falsehoods is listing CBD in a product description when there is only hempseed oil present.

Run a quick search for CBD products on Amazon.com and you'll quickly see that you find plenty of products. Currently, Amazon restricts the sale of controlled substances, which includes CBD.[31] Why then are there products touting CBD on Amazon? When you dig deeper, you will discover the product does not contain CBD at all.

A 2017 study revealed that only 31 percent of the eighty-four CBD products tested actually contained the amount of CBD listed on the label.[32]

While you're reading the ingredients, also look to see what other ingredients are present in the product. If it's a liquid, what carrier oils are used? MCT, avocado, jojoba, and hempseed oil are common carrier oils. These liquids may affect the shelf life and taste of the product.

What flavoring ingredients are used? You may find CBD products contain flavor agents like lavender, vanilla, chamomile, coffee, sugar, or peppermint. Though typically used in small quantities, each of these flavoring agents has their own properties.

If you're fighting inflammation in your body, you may want to avoid products with sugar, which is a known trigger for inflammation in our bodies.

If you are using CBD for focus and overall wellness, you may wish to avoid products containing alcohol, especially CBD-infused alcoholic beverages. CBD may amplify the sedative effects of alcohol, giving you a feeling of drowsiness or sedation. Totally not what you want if your desire is to stay sharp and focused!

However, if you are using CBD for relaxation, the calming properties of lavender and chamomile may be welcome companions. We'll be covering the wellness-related properties of herbs and spices thoroughly in Chapters 4 and 5.

EFFECTS—WHAT WILL THIS CBD PRODUCT DO FOR ME?

A CBD product label should clearly identify the intent of the product. As medical claims cannot be made on CBD products due to current regulations, often the intent is in the package design.

If you see a CBD product or advertisement that makes a medical claim like "This product prevents cancer" or "Treats COVID-19 symptoms," it is an immediate red flag! Stop and reconsider purchasing a product that makes illegal and unethical claims.

From studies and anecdotal evidence, companies know what their product may do, and they are generally creative in conveying intent on the package. A package with pastel colors, a serene sunset image, or the word "relax" on the label will generally promote a product with calming effects. Products with sleep effects often use "rest" or "nighttime" on the label. Many use dark blue colors on the label or have a moon icon on the packaging.

Again, check the ingredients to see if the products have additives like melatonin. Melatonin is a common ingredient found in CBD products formulated for sleep. Melatonin is a hormone that helps tell your body when it's time to sleep or time to wake up. This natural ingredient is something your body already produces.

According to the National Center for Complementary and Integrative Health (NIH), melatonin is an approved supplement for sleep enhancement but "There's not enough information yet about possible side effects to have a clear picture of overall safety."[33]

If you are someone who prefers to use a CBD isolate product, having other ingredients present in the product may be desirable. Combining natural terpene-rich herbs with CBD isolates can help create an entourage effect.

Additional ingredients in a CBD product may have good benefits and effects that you wish to have. You just need to consider them ahead of time and investigate each ingredient to learn more about its potential effects and side effects. Bottom line, you should always do your research and make sure you are informed about all the ingredients in any supplement, including CBD products.

ORIGIN—WHERE IS THE CBD PRODUCT GROWN AND PRODUCED?

The source of the CBD should be clear and present on the label. About thirty countries currently grow industrial hemp and/or cannabis. Kameron Norwood (cofounder of Half Day CBD) suggests that the very first question all consumers should ask is "Where is the hemp grown?"

"There's no chain of command required when imported," says Norwood. "You don't know when it was harvested, when it was grown. You can't verify if they are giving you a test if it's still current. It's a nightmare that people don't even know what they should be looking for."

If you're looking for an American-grown or sourced CBD product, the source should be clear on the label, such as a statement that reads "Kentucky grown." Even within the United States, we still need to see better standards for the growing and processing of CBD and other cannabis products. The good news is that American farmers and organizations are working diligently to improve the process.

By the time you read this line in the book, the U.S. Department of Agriculture (USDA) will likely have new standards in place and will be continuing to work on setting more. You can stay updated on USDA developments by visiting https://www.usda.gov/topics/hemp.

LAB TESTING—IS THIS CBD PRODUCT SAFE?

CBD product labels should have an easy way for the consumer to quickly obtain lab results for the product being considered for purchase. The industry standard is to include a Quick Response (QR) Code on the package.

Example:

Fun Fact: If you have a QR Code reader app, you can use the above QR Code to go directly to the website page dedicated to resource materials for Getting Baked*!*

To read a QR Code, you simply need:

- a smart phone
- a QR app for your smart phone

For most apps, you can open the app on your phone and position your phone so that your built-in camera can see the QR Code. The app then reads the QR Code and should take you directly to the third-party lab test results for the specific product you're considering.

The test results should look similar to this sample test illustration:

Sample Test

CERTIFICATE OF ANALYSIS

LAB NAME:
LAB ADDRESS:
LAB PHONE #

SAMPLE #
TEST DATE:
ISO #

CBD PRODUCT BATCH # + PRODUCT DESCRIPTION

CANNABINOID LEVELS

		Mass	Mass%
CBD			
CBDa			
CBG			
THC			
TOTAL THC		0.325	0.0325
TOTAL CBD		21.546	2.1546
TOTAL CANNABINOIDS		21.871	2.1871

MICROBIALS =   Safe Levels/PASS
FOREIGN MATTER =   Safe Levels/PASS
PESTICIDES =   Safe Levels/PASS
HEAVY METALS =   Safe Levels/PASS

Percentage of Terpenes Present (Limonene, Terpinene and so on)

FRESH-BAKED TIP: In addition to a QR Code on the product label, look for a batch number and an expiration date. These are also indicators that the company is doing its due diligence to ensure you have a quality product and consistent experience with the product.

When you look at the lab results, ask yourself:

How easy is the test to read? It should be consumer friendly.

Is the lab information easy to find? At a minimum, you should easily be able to find the name, address, and phone number for the lab that conducted the testing.

When was the lab processed? Are the lab results current? You should be able to locate the sample number and the test date.

The date should be fairly recent (within a few months for fresh product). The older the date, the longer the product has been shelved, or you may be looking at test results for a different batch of products that's being reused unethically for a new batch.

Does it look fake? Is the font the same throughout the document? Does it appear to be tampered with? Does it look like the information was altered in any way? These are all red flags of a fake or inferior report.

Does the report look like it was scanned in or is it directly from the lab source? Scanned reports are often a sign that the CBD was imported from another country. It may also be a sign that the CBD manufacturer is using the lab report from the farmer and is not conducting testing on the final product.

Can you verify the contaminants? Does the lab report include purity and safety information on the product batch?

Microbials, foreign matter, pesticides, and heavy metals should all be screened and listed as passing the test at safe levels, meaning there is minuscule (U.S. Consumer Product Safety Commission designated allowable limits) or zero presence.

If you see the letters "ND" listed on a lab report, it stands for "nondetect." This does not mean there is none of the contaminant present, it means the level of contaminant may be too low for the test to register.

Can you verify the potency? Does the lab report include the CBD and THC levels in a clear and easy-to-understand way?

For a CBD product, the CBD level should be the highest cannabinoid. THC levels should be under .3 percent (if full-spectrum) or none (if broad-spectrum or isolate). In states where CBD distillates are legally sold, the THC level may be higher than .3 percent.

Is the lab ISO credited? The ISO/IEC 17025 accreditation is applied to labs that have met "general requirements for the competence to carry out tests and/or calibrations, including sampling."[34]

What other standards does the lab have to uphold? Look for information regarding their standards and practices. Are they DEA licensed? Under the U.S. Domestic Hemp Production Program, labs must be registered with the Drug Enforcement Administration (DEA) if they are handling controlled substances, including testing hemp for THC.

You can find a listing of DEA registered labs at: https://www.ams.usda.gov/rules-regulations/hemp/dea-laboratories.

An additional standard to look for on packaging is the U.S. Hemp Authority Certified seal on products. This is a seal of approval companies can apply for to show that their products meet high industry standards, including passing third-party audits. You can learn more about this seal and how to recognize it at https://ushempauthority.org/.

PRICE—HOW MUCH SHOULD I SPEND?

Price is another important factor when you're considering a CBD product for purchase. You'll need to decide:

- what you can reasonably afford within your current budget
- what products will give you the most return on your investment

If pain alleviation is your priority, your dollars will be best invested in topical creams. Luxury bath bombs may hold great appeal to you, but at an average retail cost of $15 to $25 per bath bomb, you could easily rack up debt trying to use them daily.

CBD bath bombs can be a nice addition to your weekly regimen, and it's super easy to make your own to reduce the expense. You'll find my favorite bath bomb recipe in Chapter 9.

Jason Martin, CEO of Tree of Life Seeds (treeoflifeseeds.com) and an early pioneer in the CBD industry, also suggests looking for products that use nano-emulsification.

Nano-emulsification is the process of transforming cannabinoids like CBD into water-soluble molecules that are more readily absorbed. The smaller molecules are encapsulated to hold their form. This can be achieved in several ways, including through use of synthetics, which is currently the popular format used in the pharmaceutical drug industry.

Tree of Life Seeds products are manufactured with a four-step patented nano-emulsification that uses all-natural products. As Martin puts it, it's like "putting plant-based Spanx" on CBD molecules.

When you increase the absorption rate of CBD by the body, the product is more effective. It also means a smaller dose of CBD produced with nano-emulsification may have equal or better results than one without.

"CBD is a large molecule," says Martin. "If it's not reduced in size and processed for ideal absorption by your body, most will be wasted. Which means you have to take or use a larger dose."

Products processed using nano-emulsification may allow the customer to use less of the product. With the high cost currently attached to CBD products, using less product to achieve the results you desire equals fewer dollars spent per purchase.

Price is also a general indicator of whether the product you're considering contains CBD or not. Not all high-priced CBD products are legit, but if you see an extremely low-priced CBD product, proceed with high caution. Low prices are a red flag.

"We have an expression we use frequently, 'Friends don't let friends buy CBD at gas stations,'" says Martin. "It is buyer beware. Customers must do their homework."

Having done extensive research on this topic, I've personally found Tree of Life

Seeds products to be superior in many ways, including (most importantly) holding true to the promise of being more effective at lower doses of CBD in contrast to many other products I've tested.

I've also found Martin's buyer beware warning to be true, and have yet to see a credible product on a gas station shelf. Or at bargain basement pricing, for that matter. You're not paying more for quality CBD products because it's a fad, you're paying for the process from farm to market, which if done correctly, does have a high production cost.

This is not to say that all CBD products with a higher price tag are worth the investment. Again, you must investigate all the aspects of the company and product. But a low price tag on a CBD product is, and should be, an immediate red flag. You should proceed with extreme caution when considering the purchase. Use the information in Chapters 2 and 3 to help you out.

You should also always take into consideration the effectiveness of a product. This may mean sampling a few brands before you find the one that delivers the best results for the most reasonable cost that fits within your budget.

 FRESH-BAKED TIP: Be smart and protect your CBD investments. Proper storage of your CBD products will help them stay fresh and last longer. They should be stored in a cool place, out of direct sunlight, in an airtight container. After use, make sure to reseal the product properly before returning to storage.

CBD Package Sample

This is an example of CBD package labeling as covered in Chapters 2 and 3.

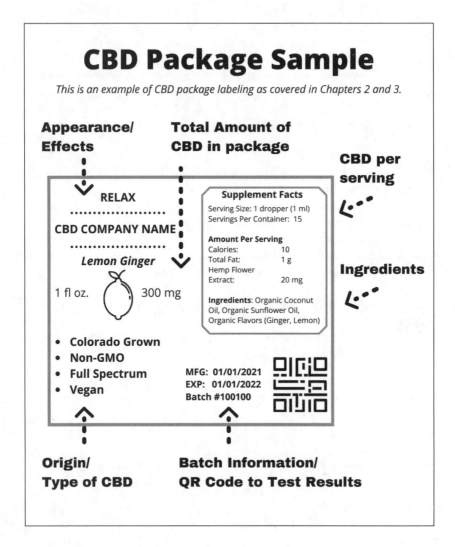

Appearance/ Effects

Total Amount of CBD in package

CBD per serving

Ingredients

RELAX

CBD COMPANY NAME

Lemon Ginger

1 fl oz.   300 mg

Supplement Facts

Serving Size: 1 dropper (1 ml)
Servings Per Container: 15

Amount Per Serving
Calories: 10
Total Fat: 1 g
Hemp Flower
Extract: 20 mg

Ingredients: Organic Coconut Oil, Organic Sunflower Oil, Organic Flavors (Ginger, Lemon)

- **Colorado Grown**
- **Non-GMO**
- **Full Spectrum**
- **Vegan**

MFG: 01/01/2021
EXP: 01/01/2022
Batch #100100

Origin/ Type of CBD

Batch Information/ QR Code to Test Results

DAZED, BUT NO LONGER CONFUSED

Whew! The world of cannabis may feel daunting, but now you are well equipped to confidently navigate the field. Josh Richman, president of Receptra Naturals (receptranaturals.com) sums up brilliantly in his company's mantra what every CBD consumer should be looking for—"easy, clear, safe."

"That's the mindset I would put out there," says Richman. "If you look at a product, you should understand within seconds what the product is and what's it's for. If you don't get that, move on. If it doesn't have a QR Code with one-click access to the report, move on. Always use some common sense here and turn to trusted resources for help."

To simplify things, note these important points:

- appearance of the product matters,
- CBD should be clearly listed in the ingredients,
- the origin of the CBD should be the United States,
- lab testing should be comprehensive and easy to understand, and
- the price should be factored into your decision-making process.

To help you out, I've created a "cheat sheet" you can use for shopping. Use this list when shopping online or in-store for your quick reference as you are considering products:

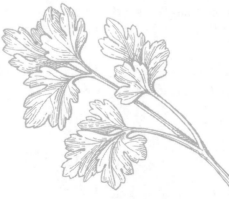

CBD SHOPPING LIST

Type: ⬤ Isolate ⬤ Broad Spectrum ⬤ Full Spectrum
        (no THC)   (no THC)   (< 0.3% THC)

Does this brand speak to me?

Does this brand address the area I need support with?
⬤ Sleep ⬤ Relax ⬤ Pain ⬤ Stress ⬤ Focus
⬤ Other: _____

Preferred dose:
(Beginner? Try starting with 10 mg CBD per serving.)

What's my budget? _____
Does this product have a price point per dose that works within my budget?

Is the product sourced and produced in the US?

Does the product have a QR code?
Does the QR code lead to clear, easily understood test results from a credible lab?

What additional ingredients are in the product?
Will they be of benefit to me?

Equally important to choosing the best CBD product option is tracking your results with each product. To get the best understanding, track your results over at least a three- to four-week period provided you have no unpleasant side effects. (As with any supplement, you should discontinue use if you have troublesome side effects and, of course, always consult your medical practitioners.)

I've included two sheets for your use:

- **CBD Product Tracker** for you to record the information about the product you purchased and quickly record daily doses and results.
- **CBD Wellness Log** designed as a journal page for use daily to record your results.

Make a photocopy of the page from this book or visit ruralmom.com/getting-baked for a download version you can print.

Whatever your style, the important point is to track your results. This will give you a clearer understanding of whether CBD is helping you with your wellness goals, if you may need to increase or decrease your dose, and any other reactions or thoughts you may have.

CBD Product Tracker

Brand:
Product Type:
Date Purchased:
Purchased from:
Dose:

Date: Date:
Dose: Dose:
Results: Results:

Date: Date:
Dose: Dose:
Results: Results:

Date: Date:
Dose: Dose:
Results: Results:

Date: Date:
Dose: Dose:
Results: Results:

Notes: _____

_____

CBD Daily Wellness Log

Date:

Wellness Goal:

CBD Dose:

Product:

Time:

Amount:

Mood (circle appropriate feeling)

Happy	Uplifted	Sad
Peaceful	Creative	Tired
Hungry	Angry	Relaxed

Thoughts: _____

_____

GETTING BAKED

Now that we've mastered the ABC's and 123's of CBD, it's time to cultivate your own medicinal garden and infuse herbal goodness into your daily lifestyle!

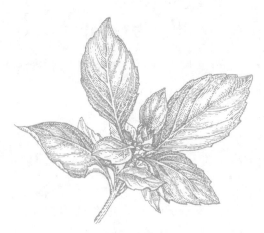

4. Get Potted
Cultivating a Medicinal Garden

Thousands of years ago, someone picked a peppermint leaf, chewed on it a bit, and said "Hey, this has a cool, refreshing taste." Eventually someone told them their breath smelled great, too.

Later, they realized that chewing on peppermint leaves made their stomach feel better and eased some of their digestive woes. And ba-da-boom! We had the first anecdotal evidence of peppermint as a medicinal herb.

According to the Merriam-Webster Dictionary, under the term "herbal medicine" a medicinal herb is defined as "a plant or plant part or an extract or mixture of these used in herbal medicine."[35]

A medicinal garden is the same as your everyday average garden, with one exception. All the plants grown in a medicinal garden are planted, harvested, and preserved with the same intent—to support your health and wellness needs.

Just like cannabis, common herbs like peppermint, rosemary, and lemon balm are chock full of terpenes and other properties that work synergistically to maintain balance within nature and within our bodies.

Also, like CBD, herbs and spices are supplements, not a substitute for good health.

You've often heard of these plant-derived substances labeled as "botanicals." This term is widely used for skin care, essential oils, hair care, and adult beverage products. "Botanical terpenes" is used to refer to isolates from plants like citrus, lavender, and cloves. Some of the most common botanical terpenes highlighted are alpha pinene, limonene, linalool, and myrcene.

Does this list look familiar?

It's because these terpenes are some of the same popular terpenes valued in cannabis plants. The more you dig in, the easier it is to connect the dots clearly between cannabis and medicinal gardening. Truly, they are a clever match in the plant world.

Used separately, cannabis plants and herbs both support your body in wonderful ways. Used together, they can often complement each other, producing even better results.

For example: using a CBD tincture in conjunction with chamomile tea can be an effective sleep aid. You might also find that common herbs may help support your body sufficiently enough to eliminate the need for other compounds like CBD. They may also eliminate the need for other OTC support aids like aspirin, heartburn relievers, or probiotics.

I rarely use antacids anymore, as I find that peppermint tea quickly alleviates my stomach troubles if I've overindulged. When I have a sore throat, a mix of thyme, honey, and lemon soothes me better than cough lozenges.

The best part—you don't need to be a certified herbalist to grow common herbs and make many simple home remedies. You just need a little herb garden know-how and a basic understanding of how to best prep and protect the health of your herbs (and spices—which we'll cover in Chapter 5).

 FRESH-BAKED TIP: Herb safety first! Before you start using any medicinal herb remedy, consult with your doctor(s) and/or other health practitioners.

If you're taking prescription drugs, it's also important to check for potential drug interactions. Speak to your pharmacist and/or doctor(s), and consult USDA resources: https://www.fda.gov/drugs/resources-you-drugs/drug-interactions-what-you-should-know.

If you have seasonal allergies, you may find you also have allergic reactions to some herbs. Even if you've never had an allergic reaction to a plant, you may still find you have an unpleasant reaction, especially when the plant is consumed in high doses or concentrated forms.

Just as with CBD, go low and slow. Start with just a few sips of a medicinal tea or a drop of tincture to assess what effect it has on your body. If you get an upset stomach, itchy skin, or any allergic reaction, discontinue use immediately.

WHAT HERBS SHOULD I GROW?

Deciding what herbs to grow in your garden is easy-peasy. Just answer these three questions:

1. What are my health concerns? _____

    _____

2. What style of foods do I like to cook? _____

    _____

3. What herbs are already in my pantry that I use regularly? _____

    _____

If you're going to grow a medicinal garden, you may as well grow your favorite cooking herbs, too!

Fresh herbs are unparalleled. Plus, you may find that some of your favorites already help alleviate some of your health concerns.

If you read my prior book, *Getting Laid: Everything You Need to Know about Raising Chickens, Gardening and Preserving,* you also know that I suggest three additional criteria for selecting plants for your garden:

1. **Choose plants that are native or best suited for outdoor gardening to your growing area.** Container gardening will give you a lot more flexibility indoors and out with herb gardening.

2. **Start with plants you are familiar with or those your neighbors have had great success with in your area.** Overwhelming yourself up front by having to tend to plants you have no familiarity with may dampen your experience.

Having a nearby resource to consult, like your neighbor, will be invaluable if you have questions or concerns.

3. **At first, grow only what you will reasonably consume or use** (for tinctures, bath bombs, hair tonics, teas, and so forth). Starting small will help you easily pay attention to what works and what doesn't. If you think you want to make one hundred bath bombs or fifty tea sachets right away, consider supplementing your bounty with organic herbs from your local farmers markets.

The great news for gardening beginners is that most herbs (and spices) do not require an experienced green thumb. When planted in the right environment, plants like basil, garlic, oregano, rosemary, and sage are relatively maintenance-free.

WHAT AILS YOU?

What are your health concerns? Are you stressed out? Need a better night's rest? Do you have dry skin? Or do you just need relief from occasional indigestion or headaches?

Medicinal garden themes maximize your efforts toward addressing your health concerns.

As we are starting small, pick your most troublesome health concern or the area of wellness you need the most support with. Then, use the following chart to help you identify herbs to consider as you plan your medicinal garden.

HEALTH NEED	HERBS THAT SUPPORT
Sleep Aid	ashwagandha, catnip, chamomile, lavender, lemon balm, lemon verbena, mint, tarragon
Digestive Aid	basil, catnip, chamomile, chives, cilantro/coriander, dill, fennel, lemon balm, lemongrass, lemon verbena, holy basil, marjoram, mint (especially peppermint) oregano, parsley, rosemary
Inflammation Reduction	ashwagandha, basil, cilantro/coriander, holy basil
Boost Immune System	holy basil, mint, lavender, parsley, rosemary, thyme
Stress/Anxiety Relief	ashwagandha, bay leaf, holy basil, lavender, lemon balm, mint, saffron, sage
Skin Care	comfrey, lavender, lemon balm, lemongrass, mint
Headache Relief	lavender, lemon balm, peppermint
Boost Mental Clarity and Focus	lemon balm, mint, rosemary, sage
Muscle Ache Relief	holy basil, peppermint
Common Cold Relief	basil, catnip, chamomile, chives, coriander, dill, lemongrass, lemon verbena, marjoram, peppermint, oregano, sage, thyme
Chronic Pain Relief	ashwagandha, holy basil

WHERE DOES YOUR GARDEN GROW?

Medicinal gardening is ideally suited for small garden spaces and container gardening. Most herbs have the same basic requirements. They need:

- access to adequate sunlight
- a nearby water source and
- sufficient soil drainage.

Some herbs (spices or edible flowers) will also need pollinators. In this case, they will need to be grown outside in a traditional garden or a container garden.

You'll want easy access to your herbs, especially if you plan to use fresh herbs regularly. Living walls, container gardening, or a raised bed garden space close to your home are ideal spots.

Great herbs also begin with great soil. Preferably, the soil you begin herb gardening with has equal ratios of organic potting soil, organic compost, and some type of material to help ensure good drainage, like coarse builder's sand.

When you grow herbs in containers, it is ideal to replace the soil once a year. For outdoor gardens, soil should be treated regularly to help restore nutrients that will be depleted by the plant. Plant rotation is also helpful.

Herb seeds are available at your local retailer or online. If you're not comfortable starting the plants from seed, you can also purchase most common herbs as seedlings or mature plants.

 FRESH-BAKED TIP: For additional gardening advice, if you are growing vegetables and fruits along with your herbs, check out Chapters 4 and 5 of *Getting Laid: Everything You Need to Know About Raising Chickens, Gardening and Preserving* by Barb Webb (Viva Editions, ISBN 978-1-63228-021-3) and visit RuralMom.com for seasonal tips.

FINDING SEEDS FOR YOUR MEDICINAL GARDEN

Heirloom seeds are wonderful for medicinal gardening purposes when you can find them. Generally, plants that originated from crops prior to 1951 get the honor of being called "heirloom."

The major difference between heirloom, hybrid, and GMO plants is that heirloom plants are the only ones that breed true. This means the same attributes (color, shape, taste, and so on) are passed on from one generation to the next. For example, if you plant an heirloom cilantro seed today and save some seeds from each subsequent crop, thirty years down the line, your children could be eating cilantro that tastes exactly the same. Also, in theory, once you've bought the original cilantro seeds for your first heirloom crop, you need never buy another pack of cilantro seed again.

It's more common to find vegetable heirloom seeds than herbs. If you do find them, make the investment! Often, they are a little pricier than other seed varieties, but you'll cherish their rich heritage and wonderful properties. Various retail mail companies, farm-store locations, and seed banks have heirloom seeds available for purchase.

The next best option is to look for hybrid seeds. Hybrid seeds were bred over time to have certain characteristics, like drought resistance. Hybrids are not GMO seeds. GMO seeds are seeds that have been manipulated using various high-tech methods in a laboratory.

Hybrid seeds are seeds from plants that are a cross-mix of two parent plants. Sometimes this occurs naturally and sometimes plant breeders manually interfere to intentionally create a hybrid. It's generally done to take the best traits of two plants and ensure the offspring (the new plant) has those desirable traits.

There's still a lot of controversy about whether all GMO plants are overall less desirable for a medicinal garden (or any farm or garden, for that matter). They've gotten a bad rep in the organic industry and from the media, but studies are still underway to determine their long-term viability and/or consequences.

I generally err on the side of not using GMO seeds for my medicinal garden, opting for heirloom or hybrid only.

Most important—prior to purchasing seeds, do your research on the company selling them. I've found the following resources to be reliable. They may be a good place for you to start when beginning your journey:

- **Johnny's Selected Seeds:** https://www.johnnyseeds.com
- **Baker Creek Heirloom Seeds:** https://www.rareseeds.com
- **Seed Savers Exchange:** https://www.seedsavers.org
- **Eden Brothers:** https://www.edenbrothers.com

GROWING HERBS FROM SEED

Beginner gardeners are often shy about growing plants from seeds, thinking they require an extra greenness of thumb. Some plants do, but when it comes to herbs, most are ridiculously easy to coax to life from seed.

Seeds can be sown directly into the garden or container. You can also start seeds inside with a seed starter kit. It's mainly a matter of preference and climate. If you have a shorter growing season, starting herb seeds inside or in a greenhouse can be highly beneficial.

An advantage of starting seeds indoors in flats or containers is that you can start them early. You also have more control over the temperature and soil conditions.

The best time to sow herb seeds outdoors is after the danger of frost has passed. Ideally, the soil should be crumbly and not too wet. It's always smart to read the back of your seed packets for any specific planting directions for your region.

You'll want to choose a spot in your garden where herbs will thrive, but not invade flower beds or vegetable gardens. While basil and tomatoes grow harmoniously together, not all herbs fare well next to flowers or vegetable plants. Herbs like mint are also quite invasive—they'll quickly take over a garden patch if you let them.

Before you plant, it's a good idea to check your soil. You can take a sample to your local extension agency and have it tested for a small fee. They'll also help make recommendations for fixing any problems so that you can ensure your soil is as healthy as can be to help nurture your medicinal herbs.

The majority of herbs love well-draining soil and sunny spots. You'll want to find a spot where it's easy to keep the soil moist but not soggy. Raised beds and container gardens work exceptionally well for this purpose.

Seeds are generally sown in furrows and covered lightly with soil. Always check the seed packet for ideal depth of seed planting. After sowing the seeds, I always press down gently on the top of the soil with the palm of my hand to assure good contact between seeds and soil.

Be sure to mark and label the rows as you're planting. Trust me, it's super easy to forget what is where, even immediately after planting your garden! It's best to mark as you go so you'll have no trouble locating everything later.

Directly after planting your seeds, spray a fine spray of water to moisten the soil to help the seed germination along. Don't soak the soil. Too much moisture can cause seeds to not perform as well and even to rot in the ground before germination can take place.

After leaves appear on your herb sprouts, thin crowded areas by pulling out the weaker plants. This will allow the hardier plants to truly flourish.

PLANTING A CONTAINER MEDICINAL HERB GARDEN

I grow many of my herbs (and spices) in containers. Most culinary herbs are fast-growing and thrive in a container garden.

Growing them in pots, rather than a garden plot, allows me to easily move them. This is very handy when the plants may need more sunlight or need to be brought inside when there's a chance of frost. It also gives me more flexibility in altering soil conditions for optimum growth, and allows me to keep plants I use daily right in my kitchen.

Herbs generally require a lot of sunlight to grow well, so if you plan to grow them inside, you do need to have a location that receives direct sunlight for the bulk of the day.

Ideal choices for containers are those made of untreated wood, clay, ceramic, stone, or food-safe plastic. The size of the container will depend upon the needs of the herb. Basil and rosemary grow tall and will generally do well in a large pot. Thyme is a short plant that cascades. Hanging planters are perfect for this herb.

Self-watering containers are a good option if you think you might struggle to find time to water your plants each day. Even if you have the time, it's a nice convenience to have. And it's enormously helpful toward maintaining optimum plant health if you're away from home a lot due to work or travel. Before choosing containers, it's always a good idea to check seed packets for suggestions on the anticipated size of the plant and space requirements.

Weeds tend to crowd traditional outdoor gardens. There's minimal need for weed control with container gardens.

Only have a small space? No problem! If you only have a small patio area or limited window space, you can use the same container for multiple plants.

If you're planning on having a window box in your kitchen with multiple herbs, place the tallest herbs in the center and the low-growing herbs on the ends. Trailing plants like oregano and thyme will then simply cascade over the sides of the planter and not crowd the other herbs.

Aromatic plants like lavender and rosemary are lovely to keep in small places, as they stimulate your senses. Rosemary is herby and woodsy, restorative, and purifying in aromatic terms. Lavender is perhaps the most well-loved herb for its soothing scent, which is said to promote peace and calm within the home.

TENDING TO YOUR MEDICINAL HERBS

When growing herbs, treat them like any other plant. Pruning and cutting back the leaves brings even more leaves.

As you cut and use fresh basil, oregano, rosemary, and thyme, they will continue to flourish. In fact, some herbs may grow faster than you can find use for them, so share some with your friends and neighbors!

Just like any plant, each herb also has a cycle, specific needs, and varied harvest requirements. I've included basic information and tips on each to help you get started on the path to success with your medicinal garden.

ASHWAGANDHA

Botanical Name: *Withania somnifera*

Cycle: perennial shrub

Ashwagandha is sometimes referred to as "Indian ginseng." You'll find over 1,000 articles on pubmed.com regarding the attributes and potential of this Ayurvedic wonder.

Container-friendly, ashwagandha grows to about three feet tall, and requires a dry spot, full sun, and rich, well-draining soil. A hearty plant, it thrives in poor conditions that other plants might not tolerate.

Special Needs: Ashwagandha needs space, so a large, deep container is preferable for optimum growth. Mix sand in the soil to improve drainage. The plant does not tolerate wet soil well.

Harvest: When berries start to form and leaves wither and yellow, it's time to harvest the ashwagandha root. Gently remove and clean the root, cut into small pieces, and dry. The leaves and berries are not used for consumption, just the root. The berries can be dried, however, and crushed for seeds for replanting.

BASIL

Botanical Name: *Ocimum basilicum*

Cycle: annual herb

One of the most popular herbs commonly found in salads, vinegars, oils, and pasta dishes, basil is a delight for the senses and palette. It's said to bring wealth to anyone who carries a sprig in their pocket, and it thrives in all types of garden settings, including container gardens.

Special Needs: Basil is highly frost sensitive. If there are frost warnings, it's best to bring basil plants inside or cover well until the danger of frost has passed.

Harvest: A well-cared-for plant will produce multiple harvests. Remove flower spikes as they appear to encourage growth. Regularly harvest fresh basil, starting with larger leaves on the outside, allowing the smaller leaves to develop further.

BAY LEAF

Botanical Name: Laurus nobilis

Cycle: perennial tree

Commonly found in marsh and swamp areas, the bay leaf has a rich history. Sweet Bay and Red Bay trees produce these lovely leaves that are found in most modern kitchens.

In ancient times, Olympian champions in Greece were honored with bay leaf garlands. Today, Grand Prix winners receive wreaths of bay leaves.

Special Needs: Bay trees are very particular about where they grow. In the United States, they typically only do well in USDA Zone 7. You can certainly attempt to grow a bay tree in a large tub as an ornamental tree, but it may be much easier, and less expensive, to simply purchase bay leaves at your local natural food store.

If you are lucky enough to live in a region where bay trees are native and grow in the wild, you may be able to forage some for use.

Harvest: The best flavor comes from mature bay leaves that are picked and dried prior to use. Bay leaves should always be removed from recipes after cooking or steeping. They are difficult to digest and can cause damage to the intestinal tract if consumed.

FRESH-BAKED TIP: The United States hardiness zones are determined by the U.S. Department of Agriculture. They are based on scientific calculations that take into consideration the average temperature in a region. This helps determine growing conditions in each area.

You'll generally find zones listed on the back of seed packets to help you determine whether the seed is ideal for planting in your area. My area in Kentucky falls in USDA Zone 6b. When I consider medicinal herbs for my garden, I aim to choose seeds that are ideal for this zone.

However, if you use a greenhouse or set up a container garden inside your home, sometimes you can coax plants outside of your zone to thrive in your area. The USDA Zone selection is not a hard and fast rule, but it is an excellent guideline to use to help ensure your gardening success.

Wondering what USDA Zone you're in? Consult the USDA Plant Hardiness Zone Map at https://planthardiness.ars.usda.gov/PHZMWeb/ to find out.

CATNIP

Botanical Name: *Nepeta cataria*

Cycle: perennial herb

We all generally associate catnip with being intoxicating to cats, but it's also a popular herbal tea ingredient for humans, valued for its digestive and relaxation properties. Drought tolerant, it's an easy plant to grow, requiring extraordinarily little attention.

Special Needs: Cats may, indeed, be overly attracted to this plant, so it's best to find a space where cats will not interact with it. I generally keep catnip in my greenhouse year-round, as I have both indoor and outdoor cats.

Harvest: Remove the top of the plant when it is in full bloom. Tea may be made from fresh or dried leaves.

CHAMOMILE

Botanical Name: *Matricaria recutita*

Cycle: annual herb

A member of the daisy family, chamomile is a beautiful plant to grow in your garden or as part of the natural landscape around your home. It's delicious, slightly fruity flavor makes it a tea drinker's favorite.

Special Needs: Chamomile loves water but not wet soil, so be sure the soil has good drainage. Mulching around chamomile plants is helpful in keeping the soil moist throughout the summer.

Harvest: Flowers and leaves may both be picked at maturity and used fresh or dried for future use. The best flavor comes from the yellow center of the daisy-like flowers, the leaves can sometimes be bitter.

CHIVES

Botanical Name: *Allium schoenoprasum*

Cycle: perennial herb

With their light onion flavor, chives are excellent when paired with just about any culinary dish. They grow quickly and are best when used fresh.

Special Needs: Chives are excellent container garden plants requiring little maintenance. When cared for well, they'll return to deliver a fresh batch of goodness each year. Divide and repot every other year for best results.

Harvest: Clip leaves throughout the growing season. Chive flowers are edible, too, but the stems directly beneath the flower may be bitter and are best removed and discarded.

CILANTRO/CORIANDER

Botanical Name: *Coriandrum sativum*

Cycle: annual herb

Some call it cilantro, some coriander—bottom line, the plant produces both cilantro leaves and coriander seeds. Cilantro's versatility, cool weather tolerance, and quick cycle boost it to the top of the spring planting calendar.

Special Needs: Cilantro prefers cool, moist soil. In hot areas or summer, mulching is a must. Plant a new batch of cilantro each month for a constant supply throughout the growing season.

Harvest: Snip leaves early in the season (after the plant has reached at least six inches in height), starting from the bottom of the plant and working your way up. Never harvest more than one-third of the plant at a time.

As the plant matures, allow it to flower and produce coriander seeds for harvesting. Harvest seeds as soon as the pods ripen.

COMFREY

Botanical Name: *Symphytum officinale*

Cycle: perennial herb

Healers have used comfrey for centuries for sores, bruises, wounds, and boils.

Part of an ideal medicinal garden first aid kit, comfrey is used topically and *never* ingested. Do not eat this plant or attempt to use it for tea—it is toxic when ingested.

Comfrey is a lovely plant producing purple bell-shaped flowers that's fun to grow even if you never have a need for it.

Special Needs: Comfrey has a deep root system, so if you're growing it in a container, it will require a large, deep one to thrive.

Harvest: Gently dig up the root, remove leaf and plant matter.

To create a comfrey compress: Clean root and cut into slices. Wrap a slice in gauze, then mash with a mallet. Dip the gauze into boiling water. Cool slightly until it is comfortable to touch, then apply to sore or bruise. Tape or bind with a cloth bandage and leave on for up to twelve hours.

Do proceed with caution as comfrey can cause an allergic skin reaction in some people.

DILL

Botanical Name: *Anethum graveolens*

Cycle: annual herb

The distinct taste and smell of dill is hard to miss! In fact, I'm told an old mountain remedy in Kentucky for curing hiccoughs is to rub a sprig of dill to release the plant oils and inhale the sweet scent.

Most often associated with pickling or salmon, the delicate leaves of the dill plant are quite powerful in flavor.

Special Needs: Dill loves moist soil. Mulching is desirable.

Harvest: Cut clippings from young plants regularly to use fresh for seasoning. Dill has less flavor as it matures. For pickling, pick dill heads before the seeds are fully formed. Cut entire plant before seeds turn brown to harvest the seeds. When harvesting, if you leave one plant, it will seed your garden for the next season.

FENNEL

Botanical Name: *Foeniculum vulgare*

Cycle: perennial herb

Known for its strong licorice-like flavor, fennel has a fern-like appearance. In folklore, fennel was used for protection to ward off evil spirits when grown around the home or hung in windows. In modern times, it's a favorite seasoning for soups, stews, and salads.

Special Needs: Fennel loves sun and moist soil. Mulching is desirable.

Harvest: Cut clippings from young plants regularly to use fresh. Remove blooms when they appear to prevent it from going to seed unless you wish to harvest the seeds.

To harvest seeds, cut entire plant before seeds turn brown.

Fennel bulbs may be used for cooking or salads, too. Harvest the bulb when it matures and reaches a size of four inches or more.

HOLY BASIL

Botanical Name: Ocimum sanctum

Cycle: annual herb

Also known as Tulsi, Holy Basil is sacred in ceremonial Hinduism. Though different from common basils, like Genovese, it can still be used in much the same manner.

Special Needs: Find a reliable source for seeds, as Holy Basil is not as common in the United States. A perennial plant in tropical climates, Holy Basil is considered an annual in the majority of the U.S. states because it is highly frost sensitive. Holy Basil may be planted after the last frost of spring and must be harvested before the first frost of fall. If there are unexpected frost warnings, it's best to bring basil plants inside or cover well until the danger of frost has passed.

Harvest: A well-cared-for plant will produce multiple harvests. Pinch off flower buds as they appear to encourage growth. Regularly harvest fresh Holy Basil, starting with larger leaves on the outside, allowing the smaller leaves to develop further.

LAVENDER

Botanical Name: Lavandula angustifolia

Cycle: flowering perennial

Used for everything from teas to crafts, lavender is a versatile plant with a remarkable fragrance. A bee-friendly plant, its fragrance also attracts humans and is generally praised for its relaxation-inducing properties.

Special Needs: Lavender is well suited for container gardens but must be brought inside for the winter in cold climates. It prefers full sun and drier soil with good drainage.

Harvest: Gather flower tops when buds begin to open to use fresh or dried. Dried lavender keeps its fragrance for several months. Leaves may be harvested for creating lavender oils.

 FRESH-BAKED TIP: Herbs can help beautify your home. Thyme is a welcome addition to any landscape because of its gentle creeping habit and wonderful fragrance. For this reason, thyme is ideal for filling in along paths and walkways. If you want a distinctive look and wonderful citrusy aroma, look for the lovely lemon thyme variety.

Sage, with its soft greyish-green leaves, is another herb that is as beautiful as it is delicious. Planted in groups, it makes an attractive focal point at the front of a landscape bed.

You may want to consider adding edible flowers such as violas and chive blossoms, as well. Tuck fragrant herbs and edible flowers in among your more traditional annual ornamental flowers.

Rosemary is a great addition to your landscape because it offers a strong vertical element. This complements plants with more compact and trailing growth habits.

LEMON BALM

Botanical Name: *Melissa officinalis*

Cycle: perennial herb

This lovely lemony plant attracts all the bees to the yard! Lemon balm is a bushy herb with fragrant leaves that are wonderful in teas or water, and delightful when added to a glass of white wine.

If you rub lemon balm onto your skin, it acts as a natural insect repellent for mosquitoes and gnats.

Special Needs: Part of the mint family, lemon balm loves to spread and enjoys moist soil conditions.

Harvest: Pick leaves before the plant flowers, use fresh or dried. Most herbs will stay fresh for at least one year once dried, but lemon balm loses potency quickly, so it's best to use within three months of drying.

LEMONGRASS

Botanical Name: *Cymbopogon*

Cycle: perennial herb

Traditionally planted around houses to repel snakes, this ornamental grass is full of citrusy flavor. Infused in water or tea, it's a mild digestive aid that's chock full of vitamin C.

A fast grower, lemongrass also reaches some high heights, so if you're container gardening, a large container on a patio deck is an ideal spot.

Special Needs: Appreciates full sun and moist soil, but lemongrass is hardy and will do quite well even if you sometimes neglect it.

Harvest: Cut long blades and use fresh or dried. The most intense flavor is in the blade part nearest the base of the plant.

LEMON VERBENA

Botanical Name: *Aloysia triphylla*

Cycle: perennial herb

Beautiful pink flowers will dot this shrub-like herb, which can grow up to six feet tall. In folklore, lemon verbena is often associated with love. Wearing a sprig or adding leaves to your bath water is said to potentially help you attract a mate.

Special Needs: Grows quickly and is a nice, sturdy plant that requires little attention. Immensely enjoys sunny locations.

Harvest: When the plant matures, harvest leaves in full and use fresh or dry. Dried lemon verbena leaves hold their scent for a long time, making it a lovely choice for potpourri.

MARJORAM

Botanical Name: *Origanum majorana*

Cycle: perennial herb

Closely related to oregano, and often called Mountain Mint or Sweet Marjoram, this herb is a fast, flavorful grower. Its flavor is stronger than oregano but can be used in all the same culinary dishes.

Special Needs: Treat in the same manner as oregano.

Harvest: After the plant is at least five inches tall, pick leaves prior to use and use fresh or dry for later use.

MINT/PEPPERMINT/SPEARMINT

Botanical Name: *Mentha/Mentha x piperita/Mentha spicata*

Cycle: perennial herb

A popular favorite among herbs, all mint plant varieties are loved for their scent and taste. Chocolate mint (my favorite variety), pineapple mint, peppermint, spearmint—they are all delightful and vary in strength of flavor.

Pick a mint leaf, rub it to release the oils, and then breathe in the invigorating scent. If you have a headache, try rubbing fresh peppermint leaves on your temples for aid in headache relief.

Special Needs: Mint grows prolifically and will produce a long season. Cut back regularly to prompt new growth. This herb spreads both above and below ground, allowing it to quickly take over a garden patch. Container gardening is ideal to prevent mint from overtaking your land.

Harvest: Use young leaves with fruit in the summer. Clip mature leaves for culinary season, teas, and for drying.

FRESH-BAKED TIP: Bee balm, also commonly referred to as horsemint or bergamot, is a large perennial in the mint family. Various breeds of this plant range in height from one to six feet and produce large blooms in the shape of fireworks.

In the medicinal world, bee balm tea is known for having a soothing effect on the digestive system. Both the leaves and flower petals can be used to create a lovely brew.

Bee balm enjoys sunny spots and well-drained soil. The plant will tolerate partial shade but will flower less and spread out more. Shade can also make the plant more susceptible to diseases like powdery mildew and rust.

If you are a nature lover, bee balm is a fabulous plant for attracting wildlife to your garden. The long tube-shaped bloom is desirable to hummingbirds and, as the name suggests, bees adore the plant (as do butterflies).

OREGANO

Botanical Name: *Origanum vulgare*

Cycle: perennial herb

A favorite in pasta dishes, pizza, marinades, and egg dishes, oregano has a full, robust flavor when used fresh.

Special Needs: Oregano is a sun lover but does best with around six hours of full sun in the morning and a bit of shade in the late afternoon. Plants prefer well-drained but moist soil, so mulching is a good option for aiding oregano throughout the summer.

Harvest: Pick leaves prior to use and use fresh.

PARSLEY

Botanical Name: *Petroselinum crispum*

Cycle: biennial herb

Beautiful, big, dark green leaves of parsley deliver a mild flavor that pairs with absolutely everything. You'll often find parsley as a garnish on a dish, rather than an ingredient, because the flavor diminishes with cooking.

Special Needs: A partial sun plant, parsley is a slow grower, especially in summer. Rather than growing from seed, it's sometimes useful to purchase an established plant for your container garden. You may also wish to purchase cut parsley from your local farmer's market to supplement your needs.

Harvest: Clip fresh daily. Harvest mature leaves from the outside of the plant first, allowing inner leaves to grow bigger. Parsley flowers in the second year. Remove all flowering stalks to continue harvesting leaves throughout the season.

ROSEMARY

Botanical Name: Rosmarinus officinalis

Cycle: perennial herb

Chock full of aromatics, a few sprigs of rosemary or a rosemary wreath in your kitchen can truly freshen and liven up the space. Legend has it that if you place a sprig of rosemary under your pillow at night, you'll have sweet dreams.

Special Needs: Rosemary thrives in sunny spots, though it fairs well in partial shade, too. It does very well in containers and as an edible ornamental in landscapes.

Harvest: Prune rosemary in midspring, use the fresh leaves. Pick leaves throughout the season and use fresh for seasoning, teas, and tinctures.

SAGE

Botanical Name: Salvia officinalis

Cycle: perennial herb

The strong flavor of sage is often found in winter holiday dishes. A sun-loving plant, sage produces velvety grayish-green leaves and pretty blue flowers in early summer.

Special Needs: Prune back below the flowers when blooming is finished. After about four years of growth, sage will need to be replaced, as the stems will become too woody.

You can keep the older sage plants as ornamentals, but for the best flavor, new sage plants will need to be established.

Harvest: Pick leaves when mature and dry for recipes and teas.

TARRAGON

Botanical Name: *Artemisia dracunculus L.*

Cycle: perennial herb

Part of the sunflower family, this mild herb is rich with potassium, manganese, and iron. Each year after planting, tarragon will return larger than the year before.

Special Needs: French tarragon is the standard in gardens, but it is a temperamental plant. If you have difficulty growing it, try Spanish Tarragon (often referred to as Mexican tarragon or Mexican mint marigold) instead. It has a slightly different flavor but all the same benefits.

Harvest: Remove leaves throughout the season when mature; use fresh. The flower petals are also edible and fun to sprinkle in salads and tea. However, the flower petals do not taste the same as the leaves.

THYME

Botanical Name: *Thymus*

Cycle: perennial herb

Small, but mighty in flavor, thyme is a savory herb that draws butterflies and honeybees to your garden with its spring blooms. After blooming, thyme will spread out and deliver an abundance of leaves.

Special Needs: Thyme grows best when planted in full sun. It also needs well drained, rich soil. After thyme blooms, prune by pulling all stems into a bunch and cut below the blooms (about a third of the way into the plant). This practice encourages new growth and develops a full, lush, plant.

Harvest: Pick leaves during the growing season to use fresh or dry for later use. You can also snip the stems regularly to shape the plant and then harvest the leaves from your snipped portions for use.

FRESH-BAKED TIP: Herbs like cilantro, oregano, mint, and dill will reseed each year if you let the plant mature. Once it flowers and seeds, the seeds will fall to the ground and you'll have a new crop the following year.

You can also harvest seeds like coriander, dill, fennel, celeriac, and mustard for seasoning, tinctures, pickling, and teas. Learn more in Chapter 5.

AN IMPORTANT NOTE ABOUT PESTICIDES AND YOUR MEDICINAL GARDEN

Don't ever use any chemical pesticides in your medicinal garden, ever.

The End.

Seriously!

Harmful chemicals on your medicinal plants equals harmful chemicals that will be absorbed by your body. That pretty much defeats your health and wellness intentions.

All medicinal gardens should ideally be grown organically. If you have weed problems, pull each weed out by hand or use a hoe to help you weed larger gardens.

If you have bug invasions, pick the bugs and bug eggs off the plant by hand. Squash the bugs and dispose of them by feeding them to your chickens or leaving them out on your lawn for local birds and bigger bugs to enjoy. Burn all the bug eggs you collect.

Other practices that discourage bug infestations are:

- spraying mature plants with a forceful stream of water
- using floating row covers or netting
- planting earlier or later in the season to avoid prime insect frenzy times
- container gardening indoors
- applying ground covers to help keep bugs from traveling across soil

Herbs can be utilized for pest control, making them a great choice for container gardening on your patio or deck.

- Mint plants (especially peppermint) repel ants, aphids, caterpillars, spiders, and more.
- Lavender, lemongrass, and mint can help keep mosquitos at bay.
- Lavender, lemongrass, sage, and thyme repel ticks.
- Basil, clove, rosemary, lavender, and mint repel flies.

To make a spray using these natural herb remedies, combine ten drops of essential oil (from one of the herbs suggested above) with one gallon of cool water. Stir to mix thoroughly. Spray on plant and soil early in the morning (right after sunrise is ideal). Repeat once per week until the problem is resolved.

Bugs pestering you in the garden while you're gardening? Use my favorite easy-to-make bug spray recipe:

- 5 drops of lemongrass essential oil
- 5 drops of lavender essential oil
- 5 drops of peppermint essential oil
- 2 tablespoons apple cider vinegar
- 2 tablespoons of water

Just mix all ingredients together, pop into a spray bottle, and spritz on clothing and gear you're wearing. Spraying essential oils directly onto your skin may cause a reaction, so I opt to spray on clothing and gear, and I find it works just as effectively.

Experiencing disease or mold symptoms on your plants? Remove affected areas of the plant. If mold is persistent, it's generally a result of overwatering. Cut back on watering and allow soil to dry between watering.

Opt to water early in the morning to give soil a chance to drain properly and plants the chance to dry off. Watering at night may cause the plant and soil to maintain too much moisture, which may encourage issues like mold growth.

If the entire plant is lost to disease, destroy the plant, and start over. It's best to burn diseased plants. Don't put them in your compost pile, as it will taint the soil and then may later spread to other areas of your garden that you use the compost mix for.

Also, always wash your tools after use to help prevent spreading disease or mold inadvertently.

JOURNAL IT!

One of the best practices you can have as a medicinal gardener is to keep a journal of your gardening efforts. This will help you to have a happy, healthy harvest every year.

It's easy to forget what went right, where you purchased seeds from, or what problems you encounter. By journaling it, you'll have a handy reference to refer to that will save you oodles of time and tons of heartache.

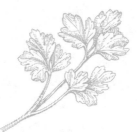

Medicinal Garden Journal

Type of Seeds:
Source of Seeds:
Date Planted:
Amount Planted:
Garden Location:
Days to Maturity:

Date: Observations/Yield: Ideas:

_____

_____

_____

_____

_____

_____

_____

_____

_____

_____

_____

_____

_____

Note: Copy this page for your use or visit ruralmom.com/getting-baked for a print-able version of this journal page.

SHOULD I GROW HEMP IN MY MEDICINAL GARDEN?

Before considering adding any cannabis plant to your garden, including industrial hemp, you need to research your state regulations. Even in states where cannabis plants are approved for recreational use, you'll likely still need to obtain a permit (typically a $100–$200 onetime fee) for growing cannabis plants in your home or on your property.

You should be able to find information on federal laws and your state's current laws and regulations on the USDA website: https://www.ams.usda.gov/rules-regulations/hemp.

The next question to ask yourself is "What do I want to use the hemp for?" Do you plant to grow hemp for seeds, fiber, oil, or CBD?

If you plan to use the plants to produce smokable CBD flowers or make hemp butter, that's very doable. If your plan is to grow hemp with the objective of producing your own CBD oil, that's more complex.

Processing and extracting CBD oil from a hemp plant effectively is expensive. This is one of the primary reasons why CBD products in the current marketplace are expensive.

CBD isolate powder can be purchased to create your own custom tinctures. You'll simply need a carrier oil to mix the isolate with, like almond oil or MCT oil. After you decide what dose you want each portion to have, you then measure the ingredients accordingly and mix the CBD isolate powder with the carrier oil until the powder is fully incorporated. This process can take a while (up to one day or more) for the CBD powder to fully infuse with the oil.

The drawback, of course, to using CBD isolate powder is that you will not have terpenes, other cannabinoids, or additional beneficial plant matter in your mix.

If you grow your own plants, it is possible to make your own full-spectrum CBD oil at home, since you will have access to cannabis (hemp or marijuana) flowers with high CBD concentrations. An internet search will reveal a variety of methods available.

Without more sophisticated machinery, it will be difficult for you to produce a refined product and to extract the full potential of the plant when creating a CBD oil at home. Plus, you'll likely not be able to produce enough for use throughout the year.

Keep in mind that most states that allow growing cannabis at home for medical or recreational purposes only allow up to four to six plants. This will limit your ability to extract the quantity and potency of CBD oil that you would need for regular use.

This isn't to say you shouldn't decide to try to grow cannabis plants and produce your own CBD oil at home. It can be a great way to connect with nature, control the source of your CBD, and supplement your CBD oil purchases, thereby decreasing the amount you may normally spend buying CBD oil from a manufacturer.

At the National Hemp Expo in Louisville, Kentucky, I attended a hemp farming session with speaker Danny Plyler, a partner at Chronic Nomad Cannabis Company (nomadchronic.com). Afterward, I had the chance to have a lengthy chat with him about growing cannabis at home.

Plyler is not only an expert cannabis grower, he walks the hemp walk in all facets of life, from treating his PTSD with cannabis products to retrofitting his diesel car to run on hemp oil. He suggests that growing cannabis at home is going to be an activity we see more and more home gardeners embracing in the future.

"Gardening itself has therapeutic value," says Plyler. "Why not teach consumers to grow their own medicine? It gives them the opportunity to save hundreds of dollars and gain beneficial results from a therapeutic hobby."

Plyler concedes that cannabis businesses are likely to grow and produce superior products, but that shouldn't stop someone from growing their own. Home gardeners can produce viable and beneficial cannabis plants.

"You have to care for a CBD plant you are growing for flowers like you do a high-end tomato plant," says Plyler. "And just like tomatoes, you have to obtain the right seeds to produce the plant you want."

Hempseeds can be purchased from dispensaries and nurseries in states where cannabis has been approved for home growing. You can also find hempseeds online and/or at health food stores, but buyer beware—these are generally sterilized seeds that will not grow when planted in soil. They are for consumption only.

Hemp is a hearty, sustainable annual plant. It grows quickly, requires less water than other plants like corn, and generally does not need much, if any, fertilizer, herbicides, or pesticides. Warm weather and well-drained soil are the basics needed to keep the hemp plant happy.

If you choose to fertilize hemp, Plyler suggests proceeding with caution. "Common fertilizers like 20-20-20 Soluble Fertilizer will make your CBD plants 'hot,'" says Plyler. "Hot meaning that higher nitrogen in the soil will increase your THC production, pushing the THC level over the legal .3 percent limit."

Plants approved for home growth via growing permits are subject to testing. In states where medical or recreational marijuana plants are legalized for home growing, the level of THC is not an issue. However, if an industrial hemp plant goes "hot" and tests above the legal THC limit, they will need to be destroyed.

FRESH-BAKED TIP: Cannabis seeds germinate quickly. Plants reach a height of twelve inches or more in about three to four weeks. It generally takes about four months for hemp flowers to mature for harvest. If you're growing hemp indoors, you can generally get three to four harvests per year.

Should you grow hemp in your medicinal garden? If it's legal in your state, you may want to consider getting a permit and giving it a go. If it's not legal to grow at home in your area yet, keep it on your radar and look to other sources for your supplement needs.

5. GET WILD
Growing Spices, Foraging, and Other Exciting Additions for Your Medicinal Garden

From seasoning dishes, to use in folk remedies, religious ceremonies, teas, beauty products, and home goods, spices have enhanced our lives for centuries with their potent flavors, wonderful aromas, and amazing medicinal benefits.

You'll find numerous studies and anecdotal information praising the health benefits of these flavorful wonders. Like CBD and herbs, spices can lend a helping hand in addressing your concerns.

Just like herbs, spices deliver exceptional flavor and aromatics. Spices like turmeric, ginger, garlic, and cayenne pepper are all remarkably easy to grow, process, and store.

Others like cinnamon, ginseng, and nutmeg are not as easy to cultivate in your home garden, but they are readily available at natural food stores (and relatively inexpensive to purchase).

WHAT SPICES SHOULD I GROW?

As you did when deciding what herbs to grow, ask yourself three questions:

1. What health concerns are you trying to address? _____
_____

2. What foods do you normally enjoy cooking? _____
_____

3. What spices do you already keep in your pantry for regular use?_____
_____

While it's easy enough to purchase spices for use from your local grocer, growing your own ensures you a steady, fresh supply.

It also gives you peace of mind in knowing you have a pure, organic-grown source to use.

WHAT AILS YOU?

What are your health concerns? Just as you did with herbs, pick your most troublesome health concern or the area of wellness you need the most support with.

Next, use the following chart to help you identify spices to consider as you plan your medicinal garden.

HEALTH NEED	SPICES THAT SUPPORT
Sleep Aid	cardamom, cayenne pepper, clove, garlic, nutmeg, turmeric
Digestive Aid	celeriac, cinnamon, ginger, turmeric
Inflammation Reduction	black pepper, cinnamon, clove, cumin, garlic, ginger, mustard, paprika, turmeric
Boost Immune System	celeriac, garlic, ginseng, mustard, onions, shallots, turmeric
Stress/Anxiety Relief	ginger, ginseng, mustard, nutmeg, turmeric
Skin Care	garlic, onion, shallots
Headache Relief	cayenne pepper, ginger, mustard
Boost Mental Clarity and Focus	black pepper, cinnamon, ginseng, saffron, turmeric
Muscle Ache Relief	cayenne pepper, clove, garlic, ginger, turmeric
Common Cold Relief	cayenne pepper, cinnamon, garlic, ginger, turmeric
Chronic Pain Relief	cayenne pepper, cinnamon, clove, garlic, ginger, mustard, turmeric

FRESH-BAKED TIP: Garlic is an old remedy for removing warts. To create a wart-fighting garlic paste, simply mash a clove of garlic, remove the peel, and place the mash on wart.

Cover with a bandage for one hour. After one hour, remove the bandage and garlic, then cleanse the area. Repeat the process daily, as needed, until the wart is eradicated.

TENDING TO YOUR MEDICINAL SPICES

Many spices are valued for their roots rather than their leaves. Some have beautiful flowers, others come to us from the vegetable plant family, and some even grow on trees!

Just like herb plants, each spice also has a cycle, specific needs, and varied harvest requirements. In the same way I did with herbs, I've included basic information and helpful tips for helping these wonders thrive in your medicinal garden.

CARDAMOM

Botanical Name: Elettaria cardamomum

Cycle: perennial herb

Chock full of strong savory-sweet flavor and fragrance, cardamom is commonly found in Middle Eastern cuisines. An immune system booster with antibacterial properties, it is also used to treat bad breath. In fact, you can find chewing gums containing cardamom as a main or supporting ingredient.

Cardamom is an expensive spice to buy, but a little does go a long way. It's definitely a plant worth trying to grow in your medicinal garden.

Special Needs: A super thirsty plant, cardamom craves a regular watering schedule. It also enjoys partial shade throughout the day and moist soil. Do mulch this plant in the summer.

Harvest: Pick the fruit when fully formed and ripe, before they are fully dried. The fruit should release from the plant easily. Dry fruit, store, and grind into powder as needed. People sometimes refer to cardamom fruit as "seeds" or "pods," but technically they are a small fruit with seeds inside.

CAYENNE PEPPER

Botanical Name: *Capsicum annuum*

Cycle: perennial fruit

Often referred to as "red pepper" in recipes, cayenne packs some culinary heat! If you don't like spicy spices, this may not be the best medicinal garden plant for you.

If you do like spicy foods, you may benefit from cayenne pepper's metabolism-boosting, heart-healthy properties. Cayenne peppers can be enjoyed fresh and whole (like other peppers) or dried for use as a spice.

Special Needs: This easy-to-grow vegetable does very well as a container plant. Cayenne pepper loves sun and well-drained soil. Be careful to avoid overwatering, and protect from cold weather by covering or bringing the container inside.

Harvest: When fully ripened, clip the whole pepper from plant to use fresh or to dry.

CELERIAC

Botanical Name: *Apium graveolens var. rapaceum*

Cycle: biennial root vegetable

Chock full of antioxidants and fiber, and high in vitamin C, this hearty root vegetable's leaves and stalks grow above ground. It looks and tastes just like celery but is known for its distinct knobby root surface.

Special Needs: Celeriac has a long growing season, so it's best to start seeds indoors in early spring. This plant is a moisture lover and will benefit greatly from mulching during the summer months.

Harvest: Look for a smooth surface on the root (bulb) with no discoloration or cracks. If the center of the celeriac root is hollow, it indicates that the plant is of poor quality. This is referred to as a "hollow heart" and typically means the soil it was grown in was too dry. Harvest root and stalks. Wash and remove rough skin, store in a vegetable drawer. Use fresh.

CINNAMON

Botanical Name: *Cinnamomum verum*

See the section "What's in Your Medicinal Pantry?" (later in this chapter) for tips.

CLOVE

Botanical Name: *Syzygium aromaticum*

Cycle: perennial evergreen tree

For centuries, clove has been burned as an incense. It's thought to remove negativity and/or negative forces from the home, cleansing the area.

The traditional culinary cloves we're accustomed to using are the flower buds picked from the evergreen clove tree. You can simply purchase them already dried at your local natural food store.

Special Needs: For most U.S. gardeners, growing a clove tree will be challenging. They need to have a tropical climate to thrive, and it takes around twenty years for the tree to mature for full harvest.

If you live in US planting zones 9b through 12, you may want to consider adding this delightful treasure to your medicinal garden landscape.

Harvest: Unopened buds are gathered before they turn pink to dry for use.

CUMIN

Botanical Name: *Cuminum cyminum*

Cycle: annual herb

Part of the parsley family, this tangy spice is popularly used in Indian and Mexican cuisines. In medicinal gardening, cumin is often used to aid with digestion, and cumin seeds always add a lovely sweet and spicy taste to teas.

Special Needs: Easy-to-grow and ideally suited for container gardening, cumin loves full sun and well-drained soil. They are sensitive to overwatering, so do give them some breathing space and allow the soil to dry out a bit between watering.

Harvest: Collect seeds when fully ripe before they are fully dry. This is generally done right after the petals of the cumin flower fall off. Dry seeds to grind for later use.

GARLIC

Botanical Name: *Allium sativum*

Cycle: perennial root vegetable

At the forefront of natural remedies, the medicinal value of garlic isn't easily ignored. Used for thousands of years, it contains allicin, a natural antibiotic, which may help strengthen your immune system and can help fight infections.

Garlic can also zap the pain away from bug bites and scrapes. Just cut a clove in half and rub the cut side onto the affected area.

There are two general varieties of garlic—hard neck and soft neck. Soft neck tends to grow better in warmer climates. They produce smaller cloves but have more cloves per bulb than hard neck varieties.

Special Needs: For most climates, garlic is best planted in midfall for harvest the following summer. The area where it is planted should be covered with straw through the winter.

Garlic is a thirsty plant. When conditions are dry, it results in smaller bulbs. This makes mulching in the summer a must to keep the soil moist and cool.

Harvest: Bulbs are ready for harvest when the garlic plant tops are brown and withered. It's best to harvest garlic when the soil is dry. Carefully remove stalks and bulbs from the soil and gently shake off dirt to use fresh.

Alternately, for storage or use later, cure garlic bulbs in a cool, dark, well-ventilated spot with low humidity. Lay plant on mesh screens or racks for two to three weeks. Tying garlic braids and hanging them is an option for soft neck varieties, too. Hard neck varieties are easier to braid after they cure.

Whether fresh or cured, to use, snip off the roots and stalks. Gently remove any remaining dirt with your fingertips or a soft brush.

FRESH-BAKED TIP: Raised beds have so many advantages, including being the ideal spot for growing garlic. Gardeners gain an easy way to control the soil conditions without spending years enriching the dirt, removing rocks, or having to worry about soil acidity and alkalinity.

Garlic loves a raised bed garden for its rich soil with good drainage, but also for the ease in controlling ground temperatures. The frame of the raised bed helps absorb the heat of the sun in the early spring, heating it up more quickly in contrast to a large garden plot.

Mulch can be used to help control the effects of frost in winter and spring and then to keep the raised bed soil moist throughout the summer months. Working in natural compost each year is easy to maintain the continued health of a raised bed.

An attractive addition to your garden, raised beds are easy to make and have plenty of advantageous features—an ideal tool you should consider using when growing bulb plants like garlic.

GINGER

Botanical Name: *Zingiber officinale*

Cycle: perennial root vegetable

The key component of holiday gingerbread, ginger can be used fresh, grated, or powdered. It's lovely when paired with all fruits, especially apples and pears.

Ginger is well-known for its ability to aid with motion sickness and nausea. When I was a child, my mom always gave us a glass of ginger ale or a cup of ginger tea when we were sick to help soothe our stomach woes. Now, I also use it for its wonderful anti-inflammatory properties, too.

Special Needs: If growing ginger in a container garden, a five-gallon bucket works well. Ginger will need room to spread out.

This plant thrives in hot, humid temperatures and loves water. If you have a greenhouse, ginger is a plant that will deeply appreciate being housed there.

Harvest: Similar to garlic, ginger rhizome is ready for harvest when the plant tops are brown and withered. Gently dig out the entire plant and dust off soil. Clip off stalks. Rinse ginger in cool water to remove remaining dirt.

You may need to use a brush to gently scrub off the dirt. It's sometimes difficult to remove dirt from the crevices between rhizomes. In this case, it's okay to break them apart and rinse separately.

Some websites will tell you to start harvesting ginger after four months of growth. This is okay to do if you live in a climate where you can't grow the plant to full maturity. Do keep in mind, your yield will be much smaller when harvesting early.

 FRESH-BAKED TIP: Ginger, cinnamon, peppermint, and chamomile are all great for use in treating gas bloating and stomach pain. If you happen to overindulge during the holidays or at a party, try drinking a cup of medicinal tea using any or a combination of these for quick relief. (You'll find instructions for making medicinal tea in Chapter 8).

GINSENG

Botanical Name: Panax ginseng

Cycle: perennial root vegetable

Container-friendly, ginseng can be grown indoors or out, but it generally takes eight to ten years to reach maturity for harvest. This alone makes it more reasonable to purchase ginseng than to grow it.

As I've never grown ginseng, I'm not the best person to address the growing and harvest needs. I decided to include ginseng in this guide because it has so many wonderful properties, it should be considered for use in many of your medicinal garden creations.

My best advice is to seek out an expert in your area who has experience with this plant if you do intend to grow it. Visit a ginseng farm or work with your local extension agent to get started.

Special Needs: Loves moist, well-drained soil that is rich with organic matter. It's also a shade lover, requiring truly little sun. In the wild, ginseng typically grows in fertile forests. If you are growing ginseng in a container, it will need to be kept in a dark spot that receives little sunlight.

Harvest: Root is dug up, cleaned of dirt and debris, and used fresh or dried.

MUSTARD

Botanical Name: *Brassica*

Cycle: perennial cruciferous vegetable

There's a lot to love about the mustard plant. The young greens are great in salads, mature leaves are terrific when cooked (just like spinach greens), and the seeds deliver that delicious condiment we enjoy on deli sandwiches, hot dogs, hamburgers, and more!

Special Needs: Mustard plants love water and it's best to use mulch or a self-watering container to prevent them from getting too dry. Lack of water dramatically increases the heat in the taste.

Harvest: Once they reach four inches or more in growth, mustard greens can be harvested regularly. Harvest one leaf at a time, working from the outside in, or clip and harvest all leaves on the plant. Either way, leave about two inches of plant material at the base of the plant to encourage regrowth. Generally, you can harvest mustard greens once per month.

To harvest seeds, allow plant to fully mature, and cut off stalks when you notice the seeds begin to dry.

PS: You'll find my favorite mustard condiment recipe in Chapter 7.

NUTMEG

Botanical Name: *Myristica fragrans*

Cycle: perennial evergreen tree

Nutmeg trees produce three delights:

- the nut seed, which becomes the spice we're most familiar with—nutmeg;
- mace spice from the extra seed covering (aril) found around the nut; and
- a fruit that encases the nut, which is often pickled.

As it's relatively inexpensive and difficult to grow in the United States (as it requires a tropical environment), it's easiest to purchase nutmeg at your local natural food store.

ONION/SHALLOT

Botanical Name: *Allium cepa*

Cycle: perennial vegetable

Heart healthy and chock full of antibacterial properties, onions add an unmistakable tang to recipes. Shallots are the smaller, milder flavor cousin of larger onions like vidalia, white, and red onions.

Raw, cooked, pickled, roasted, sautéed, powdered—there are so many ways to enjoy onions from your medicinal garden.

Like garlic, they also have antibacterial properties. Have a cut or abrasion? Rub a raw onion on it to help prevent infections.

Special Needs: The natural enemy of onions are weeds. Weed onion beds regularly to ensure they have no competition for space or nutrients.

Onions grow best in an outdoor garden but can be container gardened. Shallots will thrive the best in a container garden setting.

Harvest: Onions are ready for harvest when the tops bend over and begin to wither. Pull up the entire plant to use fresh or cure for long-term storage.

To begin curing, if the weather is dry, lay on top of the ground for a few days. Then cut off the tops and move to a dark, airy location to continue curing. (See the "Cellaring Your Medicinal Plants" section in Chapter 6 for more tips.)

PAPRIKA

Botanical Name: *Capsicum annuum*

Cycle: perennial vegetable

My first experiences with paprika were probably similar to most—as the bright pop of color sprinkled atop my mom's deviled eggs and the smoky-sweet flavor that helped make my grandmother's signature Hungarian goulash so ridiculously delicious!

I learned many years later that this wonderful spice actually comes from a type of mild pepper. When the pepper is used fresh, it's referred to as a "pimentón pepper." When they're dried and/or smoked, these pimentón peppers become paprika.

Special Needs: Grown just like any other pepper plant, it relies on sunny warm temperatures and well-drained soil to thrive.

Harvest: When the peppers turn bright red, they are mature and ready for harvest. Clip pepper from the plant to use fresh or dry the pepper to use as paprika spice. (Ideally, use a food dehydrator to dry the peppers.)

SAFFRON

Botanical Name: *Crocus sativus*

Cycle: perennial flower

A dose of saffron tea is a real pick-me-up! This bright spice comes from the center of the saffron crocus flower. As you can imagine, harvesting on a large scale is time-consuming and is part of why purchasing saffron from the market is so expensive. It takes a lot of plants to produce an exceedingly small portion, which additionally contributes to the cost.

If you're going to purchase saffron, seek out companies that are certified organic and purchase the whole dried stigmas. Powdered saffron is often adulterated with additives.

Special Needs: It takes about three years to produce flowers for harvest. Purchasing established plants from an organic nursery can help ensure viability and speed up the process a little.

Saffron crocus prefers dry, well-draining soil and cool temperatures, making it an ideal indoor container plant.

Harvest: When flowers are in full bloom, use tweezers to gather red stigmas in the center of the flower. Dry stigmas; store in an airtight container in a cool, dry, dark spot. Grind as needed for teas and recipes.

When the plant is completely done flowering, trim back all foliage. Saffron bulbs multiply each year. Dig up bulbs every three to four years and divide.

TURMERIC

Botanical Name: *Curcuma longa*

Cycle: perennial root vegetable

Popular in curries, turmeric is also often used as a saffron substitute in recipes.

Golden milk, which is a drink typically made using turmeric, coconut milk, and a pinch of black pepper, is currently a hot trend in the wellness arena. This drink is used as a digestive aid and for its potential as a weight loss booster.

Special Needs: If growing in a container garden, a five-gallon bucket works well. Like ginger, turmeric will need room to spread out. This plant thrives in hot, humid temperatures and loves water. If you have a greenhouse, use it!

Harvest: Turmeric root is ready for harvesting when the leaves of the plant wither and turn brown. Gently dig out the entire plant and dust off soil. Clip off stalks. Rinse turmeric root in cool water to remove remaining dirt. You may need to use a brush to gently scrub off the dirt.

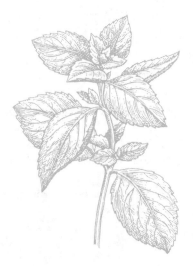

NOT JUST FOR THE BEES AND BUTTERFLIES—
GROWING EDIBLE FLOWERS

Growing edible flowers in your medicinal garden gives you lovely pops of color, a wonderful way to attract pollinators, interesting taste sensations, and some cool natural health benefits, too.

Some of the herb and spice plants you're already growing have lovely edibles flowers, like chamomile and sage.

Nasturtium (*Tropaeolum*) is an ideal plant to begin with. Similar in nature to watercress, nasturtium's sweet, peppery flavor quickly livens up salads and teas. Nearly the entire plant—leaves, buds, blooms, seeds, and pods—are all edible.

Use this chart to decide which edible flowers will support your wellness needs:

HEALTH NEED	EDIBLE FLOWER
Alleviate Stress	calendula, lavender, mustard, sage, wild rose
Lift Mood	mustard, sage, wild rose
Relieve Headache	lavender, mustard, violet, wild rose
Immune System Booster	chive, lavender, mustard, nasturtium, pansy, thyme, wild rose
Sleep Enhancer	chamomile, chive, lavender, tarragon, violet
Digestive Aid	chamomile, chive, wild rose
Inflammation Reduction	calendula, wild rose

Flowers all have a cycle, specific needs, and various harvest requirements. Some require a little extra care, but it is well worth the effort to experience the vibrant blooms.

The following tips will help you grow healthy, vibrant edible flowers in your medicinal gardening.

CALENDULA

Botanical Name: Calendula officinalis

Cycle: annual flower

A sacred herb of ancient India often used in rituals, calendula is sometimes referred to as "poet's marigold," but this plant is not the same as the popular marigold (*Tagetes*) you'll often find at seed stores.

Special Needs: A super easy grower, you can sprinkle calendula seeds in your garden and field and expect to see results. If you'd like more consistent results, start seeds indoors for transplant or container garden the plants. They do very well with a little extra pampering.

Harvest: Pick full blooms regularly for use fresh or dried. Picking the flowers (just the flower, not the stem) will encourage new blooms throughout the season.

CHAMOMILE—refer to growing/harvesting tips in Chapter 4.

CHIVE—refer to growing/harvesting tips in Chapter 4.

LAVENDER—refer to growing/harvesting tips in Chapter 4.

MUSTARD—see growing and harvest tips presented earlier in this chapter.

NASTURTIUM

Botanical Name: Tropaeolum

Cycle: annual flower

Great for use fresh or dried for seasoning, Nasturtium really brightens up your garden with lovely pops of color. To create a beautiful presentation for guests you're entertaining in your home, float some nasturtium blossoms atop teas and soups.

Special Needs: Super easy to grow, Nasturtium loves sunshine and well-drained soil.

If you don't pick the seeds, they will self-seed and spread, crowding other plants in your garden.

Harvest: Pick full flowers after bloom. Picking flowers regularly will promote regrowth.

Clip leaves as needed. Do not harvest more than one-third of the plant leaves at any time.

Harvest nasturtium seeds when fully formed before they are brittle. When fully dried, seeds can be ground and substituted in recipes for black pepper.

FRESH-BAKED TIP: Nasturtium buds and seeds can be pickled for use as a substitute for capers. They are also fun to add to charcuterie boards.

Harvest buds and seed pods when ripe on the plant before they dry out. Gently rinse and remove any dirt or debris from them. Pour buds and seeds into a four-ounce or eight-ounce mason jar* (depending upon how many you gathered).

In a small saucepan, heat one cup of apple cider vinegar along with one tablespoon of sea salt and one teaspoon of sugar. Gently stir until mixture boils. Remove from heat. Pour boiled vinegar over nasturtium buds/seeds, leaving a small headspace at the top of the jar.

Seal jar and store in a cool, dark space for two weeks. After two weeks, open and enjoy! After opening (or after two weeks of storage), store jars in refrigerator.

* Prior to canning any item, be sure to read through the "Important Canning Safety Tips" section in Chapter 6.

PANSY

Botanical Name: *Viola tricolor var. hortensis*
Cycle: annual flower

With a stunning variety of vibrant colors available for planting, pansies are a gardener's favorite. I love getting a multicolor mix of seeds so that I have pastels, jewel tones, and dual-colored flowers. Pansies are a lovely pair for infusing into honey or making flavored syrups.

Special Needs: Pansies enjoy sunshine and warm weather, making them best suited for planting in summer.

Harvest: Pick flowers in full bloom to use fresh. Picking flowers (not stems, just flowers) regularly will encourage new blooms to grow.

SAGE—refer to growing/harvesting tips in Chapter 4.

TARRAGON—refer to growing/harvesting tips in Chapter 4.

THYME—refer to growing/harvesting tips in Chapter 3.

VIOLET

Botanical Name: *Viola*
Cycle: annual flower

Flowers and leaves are edible and perfect for use in salads or as a garnish. Candied violets make a striking edible dessert decoration.

Special Needs: Excellent container plants, violets love sun and enjoy moist but well-drained soil.

Harvest: Right after bloom, remove whole flowers for fresh use.

When you pick your first violet, make a wish. Superstition has it, the wish will come true. I'm not sure if it works, as I often forget what I wished for, but it's still certainly worth a try!

Clip leaves around the flower for use fresh. It's best to not overharvest leaves. Harvest only around one-third of the plant leaves maximum from each plant to continue to encourage growth.

WILD ROSE

Botanical Name: *Rosa*

Cycle: perennial flower

Modern roses generally do not have as strong a fragrance as a wild rose. Wild roses also have an edible fruit referred to as "rose hips" that's often lacking in highly curated varieties. Both properties make wild roses the ideal choice for medicinal gardening or use in bath and beauty products.

Heirloom rose varieties known to produce rose hips are good options, as well. Aside from having a lovely fragrance, rose scent is good for lifting your mood and calming your mind.

Special Needs: Rose Carolina, often referred to as a pasture rose, is a great variety to begin with. It's a low-growing shrub-like variety that's relatively easy to grow. Just be sure to give it a sunny spot and well-drained soil.

Harvest: Wild roses are best harvested in the morning, in spring or early summer, right after bloom. Clip branch with flowers on it. Pull off rose petals for use fresh or dried.

Trim off the white or yellow strip at the bottom of each petal to avoid bitterness in taste, especially if you're brewing rose water (recipe in Chapter 8). If you're just using the petals for bath water (or other bath/beauty products), you can skip this extra step.

Rose hips are picked in the fall when they mature. To harvest rose hips, simply pick from branches to use fresh or dry. There's no need to clip branches to harvest rose hips. Split open hips and remove seeds before use.

WHAT'S IN YOUR MEDICINAL PANTRY?

In addition to growing your own herbs and spices, you'll want to stock up your pantry with supplement staples for use in creating medicinal teas, bath and beauty aids, tinctures, and recipes.

Every well-stocked medicinal pantry typically contains:

Cinnamon—you'll notice we didn't cover growing cinnamon in the "Tending to Your Medicinal Spices" section. It's rarely grown in a home setting, as it's an evergreen tree that thrives best in areas like the West Indies. Organic cinnamon is super easy to obtain for a low cost at your local health-food grocer.

Honey—touted as an immune booster, honey is handy to have for teas, cough syrups, and elixirs.

Extra-Virgin Olive Oil—used for salad dressings, cooking, marinades, and tinctures.

White Vinegar/Apple Cider Vinegar/Wine Vinegar/Brown Rice Vinegar—handy for salad dressings, marinades, pickling, tinctures, and for bath and beauty do it yourself (DIY).

Clear Vodka (or Rum)—useful for making extracts and essential oils.

Organic Cane Sugar—for use in sugar scrubs, pickling, marinades, and salad dressings.

Almond Oil—used for making bath and beauty products.

Vanilla Beans—for scent and flavoring in cooking and for creating bath and beauty products.

Dark Chocolate and Cocoa Powder—chocolate is known as a mood enhancer, but it always brings joy to your taste buds when creating edibles and smoothies.

Hempseeds—shelled seeds of hemp plants are chock full of magnesium, manganese, protein, and essential amino acids. They help build up the immune system, aid digestion, and add a lovely subtle nutty flavor to salads, smoothies, muffins, oatmeal, and more.

Sea Salt—used for cooking, pickling, bath salts, and marinades.

DIY FIRST AID KIT

There are some plants that are handy to have in your medicinal garden inventory, not necessarily for making tinctures or teas, but to aid with common ailments like sunburn, common colds, or blisters.

Aloe vera (*Aloe barbadensis miller*) is at the top of our list for its amazing properties. In folklore, this is considered a protective plant and is thought to drive away evil and protect the home where it's planted.

I first discovered the miraculous aloe vera plant when I was seven years old, visiting my grandmother in Florida. Like most fair-skinned Irish Americans, I got sunburned quite quickly after visiting the beach.

When we returned to her house, my grandmother took a leaf clipping from her aloe vera plant, split it open, and rubbed the sticky liquid gently over my sunburn. I vividly remember the instant cooling sensation and how the plant left (what my grandmother referred to as) "plant boogers" on my skin. This memory never fails to bring me heart smiles!

Aloe vera, indeed, aids with sunburn, heat burns, skin irritations, and rashes, and even in healing scars. To use, you simply clip off a tip from one of the mature leaves, squeeze the juice and pulp out, and use it just as you would any other salve.

After you clip the plant tip, the plant will naturally heal itself and continue to flourish.

Aloe vera loves sun, thrives in dry soil, and needs little water. In fact, it's a plant you can regularly neglect, and it will still produce the relief you need.

As we already discussed, **garlic and onions** are great for your first aid kit, too. Their antibacterial properties will help keep wounds from getting infected.

Lavender tinctures work well on bug bites, rashes, and skin irritations.

Holy basil or peppermint tinctures can help alleviate muscle pain.
Two drops of thyme essential oil mixed with eight ounces of water can help alleviate sore throats (and can also be used as a mouthwash to aid with sore teeth or gums).

Elderberry extracts are also good for aiding sore throats and coughs due to allergies or upper respiratory infections. You can typically find plenty of great tinctures available at your local natural food store.

As featured in the herb section, **comfrey compresses** can aid in healing sores and bruises.

Ginger capsules (you can purchase OTC or DIY your own) are great to travel with for quick aid in dealing with motion sickness and nausea.

And of course, **CBD-infused salves** are a great first aid addition for muscle pain and inflammation relief. You'll find my favorite DIY CBD salve recipe in Chapter 9!

FORAGING—A' HUNTING WILD WEEDS, WE GO!

The Blarney Castle in Ireland has a gorgeous poison garden, which to me held much greater fascination than kissing the stone!

Needless to say, I spent quite a bit of time milling around, and was surprised to find cannabis among the wolfsbane and mandrake. (Personally, I think that's all just part of the continued agenda to condemn marijuana use...)

However, the real spellbinding part of visiting the attraction is the reminder of how reliant our ancestors were on foraging the land to aid with their common ailments. There's also a lesson to be learned in taking care when foraging, as you may inadvertently stumble upon a toxic plant.

In recent years, foraging has become a popular activity. So much so that American ginseng is in danger of becoming extinct due to overforaging. Because of this, American ginseng farming is something I've been considering. If this is of interest to you, an excellent resource to begin with is *The Forest Farmers Handbook* by Rural Action and United Plant Savers (https://unitedplantsavers.org/the-forest-farmers-handbook).

There's plenty of great medicinal plant matter out in the wild, like huckleberry leaves, which are good for circulatory issues, and mushrooms, which are immune boosters high in potassium and niacin. We're all familiar with a super prolific wild grower—dandelions!

Some homeowners view dandelions as a nuisance, but these lovely flowered weeds are bumblebee, butterfly, and bird food havens. A dandelion is also an edible human food source. Everything from the flower to roots is edible. Dandelions have been used in traditional medicine by Native American, Asian, and European herbalism practices for centuries.

Other edible flowers that are fun to forage are wild roses, honeysuckle, and goldenrod (which makes a wonderful tea).

My husband loves to pluck honeysuckle every time he sees it and enjoy the sweet nectar. Sadly, the scent triggers my allergies, so it's not a great option for me.

The things I most love to forage on our little patch of land are black walnuts, wild blackberries, wild onions, and wild garlic. We also have pawpaw trees (native to the United States and found in abundance in Kentucky), but I have yet to luck out and pick the fruit before the wildlife claims it.

I'm highly familiar with all these plants, and I've gotten quite good at finding other edibles like field mustard, mayapple, violet, and pokeweed. But just because I can identify them doesn't mean I want to attempt to use them without the aid of an expert botanist or herbalist.

Many plants can be deadly. For instance, apart from the early shoots of the plant, pokeweed is poisonous. If mayapple isn't completely ripe when consumed, the fruit can be toxic. Lily of the valley, which can easily be mistaken for wild onion in early growth, can be fatal if consumed. Various nuts and mushrooms are dangerous, too.

When foraging, use extreme caution. It's never a good idea to venture out on your own.

Go with an expert you trust and even then, proceed with caution. You may still find you have allergies to some wild plants. It's also possible that the plant you forage is contaminated with animal matter, soil, or pesticides sprays that drifted over from local farms.

Try to stay in areas where you have cell phone service, and it's prudent to have your local poison control center's phone number programmed into your phone. The National Capital Poison Center Poison Control number is 1-800-222-1222 and the website is https://www.poison.org/.

My goodness! If it's so dangerous, why talk about it?

We're discussing foraging because it's a viable option for supplementing and enhancing a medicinal garden. Heading out into the wild with an expert botanist or herbalist is a highly valuable experience.

One of the foraging items you might ask them to start your education with is nuts (provided you don't have a nut allergy). Nuts like black walnuts, pecans, and walnuts can be foraged. Pine nuts from the pinyon pine are fun to find, too. They can be roasted for garnishing hummus or using in salads.

Nuts are natural energy boosters. They are typically high in fiber, which is good for your digestion, and most contain protein, magnesium, and vitamin E.

Always pick nuts from the ground, not from the tree. Gather, dry, and allow the thick hull to split. Black walnut hulls are very thick and need to be crushed. We always drive our cars over them repeatedly to get the tough hulls off!

To cure nuts, dry in shells for a month. Use an old door or window screen and lay the nuts out atop the screen to dry. Find a well-ventilated but dark spot and allow them to fully dry before storing. Sunlight degrades nuts. Always store them in their shell in a dry, cool, dark space in open containers or a basket.

Use foraged nuts for nut milk, nut butters, salads, smoothies, or simply enjoy them by the handful as a treat.

Or enjoy my favorite black walnut pesto recipe, which also makes great use of your extra basil. It can be used in the same manner as your traditional pesto made with pine nuts.

BARB'S BLACK WALNUT PESTO RECIPE

- 2 cups fresh basil leaves
- 1/2 cup freshly grated Parmesan-Reggiano cheese
- 1/2 cup extra-virgin olive oil
- 1/3 cup black walnuts (hulled, shelled, and dried)
- 3 garlic cloves
- Pinch of salt and pepper, to taste

Using a food processor, add basil, garlic, and black walnuts. Pulse until finely chopped. Add Parmesan-Reggiano cheese. Pulse until cheese is fully distributed. Scrape sides of food processor with a spatula.

Add olive oil. Add a pinch of salt and pepper. Run food processor at low speed until olive oil is fully incorporated. If the pesto is too thick and clumpy, add additional olive oil one tablespoon at a time until smooth.

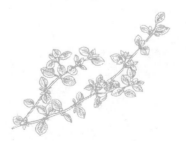

6: GET CURED

Preserving Your Medicinal Bounty

Now that your medicinal garden is flourishing, you need to figure out a plan for preserving your herbs and spices. Fresh is normally best, but the ultimate goal is to find ways to keep your medicinal plant bounty around for use throughout the entire year.

All plant preservation has four requirements for success:

- proper equipment
- quality produce
- adequate storage space
- clear labeling (including date processed and name of plant)

Avoid using herbs, spices, flowers, or plants that are diseased, bruised, molded, have insect damage, or are otherwise showing signs of rot or deterioration.

All dirt and debris should be removed from the plant prior to preserving. A light rinse may be necessary to remove any fine dirt particles.

Ideal preservation methods for medicinal plants are cellaring, freezing, pickling, alcohol curing, vinegar, oil, and drying.

STOCKING YOUR MEDICINAL KITCHEN

The success of processing an abundant harvest begins with good equipment. It's important to stock your medicinal kitchen well prior to preserving. Sure, there are items that can be used in a pinch, but inferior equipment or ad hoc substitutions could taint your efforts, producing a less-than-desirable end result.

These are the basic items you should consider having in your medicinal kitchen:

- **cheesecloth**—for straining fine particles.
- **mesh strainers**—a small fine mesh and a larger standard mesh strainer are both useful for many purposes, including rinsing and/or washing herbs.
- **drying racks**—there are specialty herb drying racks available for purchase, but standard cookie sheets work well, too. Look for cookie sheets with a grid pattern as they work best. Optionally, old window screens are handy to have for drying large harvests. Just be sure to clean them thoroughly before use.
- **dedicated towels or paper towels**—useful for catching herb seeds and leaves when drying on a rack. If you are using standard kitchen towels, it's best to keep a few thin ones set aside for the sole purpose of use in herb/spice drying. They may get stained over time from natural plant material. Towels are also helpful to have for patting off excess moisture from herbs/spices after rinsing them.
- **dehydrator**—if drying herbs and spices is part of your long-term preservation plan, investing in a quality dehydrator is prudent. Ranging in price from $50 to $500 (depending on your needs), they offer the best air circulation and drying method available for those who have high-volume or high-frequency drying needs.
- **herb scissors**—these are optional, but I highly recommend considering purchasing a set. They chop herbs quickly with a multblade system.

- **glass jars**—mason jars work very well for liquid preservation as well as dry. You'll want to have various sizes for various needs. Sizes range from four ounces to thirty-two ounces. Think about your main needs when stocking up. Four-ounce jars are great for storing dried herbs and powdered spices. Eight-ounce jars work well for storing some tinctures and tea mixes. Twelve-ounce jars and above are ideal for pickling or infusing water with herbs.
- **lids, rings, and seals for jars**—if your mason jars do not include these items, they may be purchased separately or in kits.
- **specialty glass jars**—optionally, consider purchasing items like glass oil vessels for custom oils and vinegars or amber glass dropper bottles for essential oils and tinctures.
- **measuring cups and spoons**—a set of cups ranging from a quarter cup to one full cup is sufficient. For measuring spoons, a complete set that includes a full range of sizes including an eighth of ateaspoon and two tablespoons is ideal.
- **small and large funnels**—incredibly useful for filling jars.
- **ladle**—a sturdy ladle, ideally with a small pouring lip built in, is a dream tool for ladling hot liquid into jars.
- **herb/spice grinder**—there are specialty grinders available, but you can use a simple coffee grinder. Just be sure to dedicate it for use with herbs and spices. If you regularly grind your own coffee at home, you will want a separate grinder for coffee and another for your herbs and spices to avoid cross-contamination and tainting flavors.
- **mortar and pestle**—for use in grinding spices in small batches.
- **silicone ice-cube trays**—this simple item can be used in many ways, from aiding in freezing herbs to portioning butters to sorting herbs for tea mixes.
- **freezer containers**—freezer-safe storage vessels are best for storing frozen herbs long term.
- **freezer vacuum bags**—optionally, a vacuum seal system is ideal for long-term preservation. Removing the air from freezer bags and

containers will help preserve the integrity of each item. Do consider purchasing a system for use in your medicinal kitchen if you don't already have one for your general food preservation needs.

- **food labels and kitchen storage pens**—to record the name of the product, ingredients, and the date it was made on your containers.
- **tea bags and/or tea strainer**—if you'll be adding teas to your regimen, these are necessary items to own. Tea bags are also useful for creating sachets. Tea bags and tea strainers can be useful in adding herbs to your bath rituals, as well.
- **tea kettle or pot**—again, if you're adding medicinal teas to your regimen, these are extremely helpful tools. You can also use tea kettles to help boil water for quick pickling.
- **stainless steel bowls**—stainless steel is the ideal material when working with herbs and spices. Porcelain bowls are also an acceptable option. Don't use plastic bowls—they generally absorb materials and will quickly become stained.
- **loose weave baskets**—if you're storing items like onions and garlic, a variety of loose (or open) weave basket sizes will be handy to have on hand.
- **burlap or mesh bags**—optional for storing medicinal plants after harvest, like onion and garlic.

Once you get started, you'll find plenty of enticing products available, like fresh herb keepers for the refrigerator or specialty herb jars with shaker caps. Some are worth taking a second look at—I have several fresh herb keepers for my refrigerator and they do help fresh herbs stay vibrant longer—but, when you're just getting started, you may wish to keep your investment minimal until you fully decide if medicinal gardening is for you.

As you're stocking your medicinal kitchen, take time to decide on and resolve your space requirements. When drying large batches of herbs without the aid of a dehydrator, you'll need a large area with good air circulation and no (or low) light. Light is the enemy of herbs and spices, degrading their potency.

You will need adequate space to store your preserved goods, too. Dried goods and tinctures require a cool, dark spot to rest, which will aid them in longevity of usefulness.

If you're freezing herbs, you'll need adequate, dedicated space to store them, so that they have proper airflow and do not get buried and forgotten.

IMPORTANT CANNING SAFETY TIPS

If you read my prior book, *Getting Laid: Everything You Need to Know about Raising Chickens, Gardening and Preserving*, some of the information we're about to cover may seem familiar to you. It absolutely bears repeating, since following safety guidelines while using canning preservation methods is vital to your health and wellbeing. If you're new to canning, of course, this is a must read!

With medicinal gardening preservation, you will be using alcohol and vinegar curing techniques. They use some of the same equipment, like mason jars, but differ from traditional canning methods as they do not require boil-water processing or steam-pressure processing.

Sometimes you will hear alcohol curing or vinegar curing referred to as "quick canning" or "quick pickling." The term "quick" also implies that you will be consuming the products within a short time frame, generally within one to two weeks of opening after infusing. Ideally, quick canning tinctures or foods should be refrigerated after opening, as well, to help prevent any degradation of ingredients.

The biggest health concern with any form of canning is botulism, a poisonous toxin caused by the germination of botulism spores. Botulism spores are a naturally present substance in our environment. Following proper canning techniques will destroy botulism spores and toxins.

The CDC offers a comprehensive reference guide for botulism that includes signs of, symptoms, and prevention at cdc.gov/botulism/index.html. I recommend you familiarize yourself with botulism prevention before trying any kind of canning.

When canning in any form, these techniques will help avoid potential food spoilage:

- Canning jars, lids, rings, seals, and equipment should always be thoroughly cleaned, sterilized, and dried prior to use.
- Canning jars, lids, rings, seals, and equipment should be checked for cracks, flaws, or repairs prior to use. Issues should be addressed, or the item discarded, if the flaw cannot be corrected.
- Herbs, spices, and other produce should be inspected for signs of spoilage, disease, or insect damage prior to canning. If minimal, remove blemished spots. If prevalent, dispose of foods properly. Only use ripe, disease-free, insect-free, and otherwise spoilage-free foods for canning.
- Check altitude considerations, as it can make a difference in food preservation. Consult the National Center for Food Preservation (nchfp.uga.edu) for conversion charts to ensure food safety standards are met.
- Only pure, unadulterated vinegar and alcohol should be used in alcohol curing or vinegar curing. Alcohol must be eighty proof or above.
- The canning work area and all kitchen tools (such as knives) should be cleaned, sterilized and dry prior to use.
- After filling, canning lids should always be sealed tightly to keep air out during the infusion process.
- Prior to storing, jars should be cleaned of any residue and checked to make sure the seal is tight.

If at any time, the canned goods show any sign of spoilage, look strange, or smell strange upon opening, the goods should be properly destroyed and not consumed. It's not worth the risk to consume if you think the canned goods are tainted.

If you suspect your canned goods are spoiled, do not feed to animals or compost. The canned goods should be burned or hard-boiled, cooled down, and then discarded as standard waste.

To ensure you have the best possible canning experience and knowledge base, I highly recommend downloading and reading the USDA Complete Guide to

Home Canning (nchfp.uga.edu/publications/publications_usda.html). This guide will serve as an excellent resource and provide you with oodles of additional recipe inspiration, too.

TIME TO PROTECT AND ENJOY YOUR EFFORTS!

Before you begin to preserve your medicinal garden goods, you need to decide what you will be using each herb for in the future.

Do you want to make medicinal teas? Are you ready to try using a medicinal tincture daily? Will you plan to use herbs in your beauty or bath routine? Do you want to reserve some of your herbs for cooking?

For most purposes, drying herbs/spices is a safe route to go. Some medicinal plants do not dry well, though, and are better preserved using a different method. Consult the following chart to help you determine which method will be best for each plant.

You can certainly opt to preserve your medicinal plants in a way that's not indicated on this chart—this is just a suggestion of the ideal ways to preserve the plants for maximum flavor and benefit.

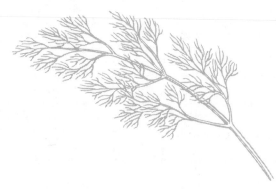

PLANT	BEST METHOD(S) OF PRESERVATION						
	Cellaring	Freezing	Pickling	Alcohol curing	Vinegar curing	Oil	Drying
Ashwagandha	X	X					X
Basil		X		X	X	X	X
Bay Leaf		X					X
Cardamom							X
Cayenne Pepper		X	X			X	X
Catnip							X
Celeriac		X					X
Chamomile				X	X		X
Chives		X				X	
Cilantro		X		X	X	X	
Clove							X
Comfrey							X
Coriander			X				X
Cumin			X				X
Dill		X	X		X	X	X
Fennel		X					X
Garlic	X		X		X	X	X
Ginger	X	X					X
Ginseng		X					X
Holy Basil		X		X	X	X	X
Lavender		X		X	X	X	X
Lemon Balm		X		X	X	X	X
Lemongrass		X		X	X	X	X
Lemon Verbena		X		X	X	X	X
Marjoram		X		X	X	X	X
Mint		X		X	X	X	X
Mustard			X				X
Nutmeg							X
Onions/Shallots	X		X				X
Oregano		X		X	X	X	X

PLANT	BEST METHOD(S) OF PRESERVATION (cont.)						
Parsley		X				X	X
Paprika		X	X			X	X
Rosemary		X		X	X	X	X
Saffron							X
Sage		X		X	X	X	X
Tarragon		X		X	X	X	X
Thyme		X		X	X	X	X
Turmeric	X	X					X

 FRESH-BAKED TIP: Prior to preserving, dirt and any other residue needs to be removed from the plant. Most herbs and spices should be washed in cold water. A colander is the perfect tool for this task because the water can drain out the bottom to help the plant dry quickly. For stubborn dirt on roots, a potato scrubber works well to help dislodge and remove it.

CELLARING YOUR MEDICINAL PLANTS

Likely, in your modern home or apartment, you don't have a cellar. Any cool, dry, dark space with good air circulation will do. A pantry, basement, or spare bedroom (with the shades drawn) are good alternatives. A bathroom, hallway, closet, or other confined, well-lit, or high-moisture space in your home are generally not good options.

Onions, shallots, nuts, garlic, and root spices will keep well in a cellar-like space.

Prior to cellaring, all dirt should be gently knocked off the plant. It's best not to wash onions, shallots, nuts, garlic, or root spices prior to cellaring. You can easily remove skins and shells or clean the plants thoroughly later, prior to preserving in any other method or prior to using for cooking purposes.

Cellared items should always be stored in open containers with good airflow, such as loose weave baskets, burlap bags, or mesh bags. Garlic is often braided and hung from a post or ceiling.

If you are using loose weave baskets, you may want to place them atop a drying rack to provide better air circulation for the bottom of the basket. This will help prevent rot from occurring at the bottom of the basket if any moisture is present.

Burlap bags and mesh bags, ideally, should also be placed atop a drying rack or hung from a ceiling or beam so that air flows around the entire bag.

Cellared items will typically last from three months to one year, depending upon the plant. Most garlic and onions, when cured properly, can easily be stored for six months. Nuts can easily last over a year when dried properly and cellared.

It's always a good idea to check in on your cellared items monthly to look for any signs of deterioration, mold, or soft spots (in garlic, onions, and other root/bulb plants). If you notice any signs of deterioration, discard affected produce and make plans to use the rest of the items soon, or consider converting healthy plants to alternative storage methods such as dehydrating or canning.

FREEZING YOUR MEDICINAL PLANTS

If you have freezer space to dedicate, many of your herbs and spices with thank you for it!

For best results, your medicinal garden herbs and spices will need to be stored with temperatures maintained at or below zero degrees Fahrenheit.

Some herbs and spices do not freeze well. Garlic is one. If you freeze garlic, it will change the taste of it, often causing the taste to be bitter. Do reference the chart included in this chapter to know which medicinal plants are best preserved frozen and which ones are not.

Root spices like ginger and ginseng can be stored fresh in the freezer. Simply place them in a moisture-proof freezer-safe bag or container, and label them with waterproof ink. Remove and grate, as needed.

Cayenne pepper and paprika may be stored whole in the freezer for later use, too. Place them in a moisture-proof freezer-safe bag or container, labeled with waterproof ink. Use within six to eight months for recipes.

Herbs like lemongrass and chives can be frozen whole. Simply put them in moisture-proof freezer-safe bags (or vacuum seal bags) for later use.

Leafy herbs like basil and cilantro do not freeze well, but they can be stored in the freezer using an ice-cube herb method. Ice-cube herbs are great for infusing water and iced tea in the summer months, adding to smoothie packs, soups, or stews, and defrosting for use in sauces or marinades. This method does not work well for recipes like pizza or pasta (unless you're using the herbs to create pizza or pasta sauce).

HOW TO MAKE ICE-CUBE HERBS

To create ice-cube herbs you will need:

- fresh herbs
- filtered water
- ice-cube trays (silicone works best, as it's easy to pop cubes out once frozen without breaking or cracking the cube)
- chef knife or herb scissors

Gently rinse and clean herbs to remove any soil or debris.

If you are planning to use the ice-cube herbs in a drink, leave the leaves whole, as they'll be easier to remove from the glass later after the ice thaws. Otherwise, using your chef knife (or herb scissors), finely chop herbs.

Fill ice-cube tray compartments with herbs.

Note: If you place exactly one tablespoon of fresh herbs in each ice-cube compartment, it will be easier for you to quickly measure out how many cubes you need for a recipe. One tablespoon of frozen herbs will equal about one teaspoon of dried herbs called for in a recipe.

If you simply plan to use frozen herb ice cubes for drinks, there's no need to measure out quantity—fill as desired.

Once all ice-cube tray compartments are filled with chopped herbs, add just enough water to each compartment to bring the herbs level with the tray edge. Place ice-cube trays on a flat surface in the freezer and freeze. I generally allow trays to freeze overnight and then complete the next step the following morning.

Remove herb ice cubes from ice-cube tray. Store in freezer-safe bags for use, when needed.

For use frozen, remove from bag and place directly into your cup of iced tea or your soup. To thaw cubes for use, use a fine mesh strainer to catch herbs as the ice melts.

This ice-cube method also works very well with edible flowers. Instead of chopping the flowers, simply place whole flower blooms or petals in the ice-cube tray compartments, cover with water, and freeze.

Rose petals, whole pansy flowers, and lavender flower bits are my favorites to make into ice cubes—they look stunning when you pop the floral ice cube into a glass of water or lemonade. Especially wonderful to "wow" your guests with!

It's also a great way to preserve rose petals for later use for your fresh rose water drinks (see recipe for rose water in Chapter 8).*

If you plan to use ice-cube herbs in soups or stews later, instead of using water, you can substitute broths (*like vegetable, chicken, or beef broth*). When you use the broth cubes in a recipe, the broth will instantly add additional flavor to your dish.

If you plan to add the ice cube herbs to marinades or dressings later, swap the water for olive oil. Then you can simply thaw and use the oil-coated herbs in your dressing without having to strain any water from the herbs.

---

* Make sure that you're never using rose petals that have been treated with pesticides, fertilizers, or other chemicals.

HOW TO MAKE FROZEN HERB PASTE

Another easy way to freeze herbs like mint, chives, cilantro, parsley, oregano, and basil is to make a paste and freeze it for later use. You'll also make good use of your silicone ice-cube trays for this method.

To create herb paste you will need:

- fresh herbs
- extra-virgin olive oil
- food processor
- silicone ice-cube trays
- multipurpose silicone spatula

Add fresh herbs to food processor. Pulse three to four times (or until herbs are coarsely chopped).

Add a little drizzle of olive oil. Puree herbs with olive oil to form a thick paste.

If the mixture is too dry (you notice all the herbs are not sticking together well), add a little bit of olive oil and puree again, repeating until mixture fully forms a thick paste.

At this point, you can simply scrape out the herb paste from the food processor and transfer to a freezer safe bag or container, then freeze. When you need the herbs, break off a chunk for use in recipes.

I find that a much easier and more reliable method is to portion the herb paste into the compartments of a silicone ice-cube tray. Again, I use one tablespoon measurements, as one tablespoon of fresh herb paste will be about the equivalent of one teaspoon of dried herbs called for in a recipe.

After you portion the paste into the ice-cube tray, place the ice-cube tray on a flat surface in the freezer and freeze overnight.

Once frozen, remove herb paste ice-cubes from ice-cube tray. Store in freezer-safe bags for use, when needed.

To use, simply pop out an herb paste cube and add it directly to your saucepan, soup, stew, or other recipes. (Don't worry if your recipe doesn't call for olive oil, the little bit of oil in the herb paste will not be problematic in most recipes).

DRYING YOUR MEDICINAL PLANTS

Fresh is generally best but drying is an excellent alternative for most herbs and spices. For herbs, drying is best for most leafy herbs. Exceptions to this rule are basil, dill, parsley, tarragon, and chives. Drying often changes the flavor profile of these five herbs and can quickly diminish their potency. You certainly can use dried versions of these herbs—in fact, you probably see them on store shelves regularly. This doesn't mean it's an ideal preservation method, it's merely a convenient one for manufacturers of these products.

To begin the drying process, gather herbs at peak growth, prior to bloom. Always keep in mind that light and heat will fade plants and diminish flavor.

Herbs can be dried in many ways. The first, and easiest, method is to lay the herbs on a drying rack. Place the stalk and leaves flat on a mesh screen, with paper towel underneath the screen (to catch small leaves). If you only collect the leaves without the stalk attached, lay the leaves on the drying rack in the same manner.

The drying rack will need to be placed in a dark, dry area with good air circulation.

Alternatively, herbs can also be dried in bunches. Tie them with a string at the stalks and hang them leaf side down. Herb bundles can be hung on a nail that protrudes from the wall or on a clip fastened to a clothes line (or any other innovative way you can think of that ensures the herbs have adequate air flow).

This can be done indoors or out. If you have a barn, it can be an ideal spot to dry herbs in this fashion. If the humidity is high outside, though, it will not yield an ideal result, as the herbs will maintain too much moisture. You may also be inviting bugs or other pests to disturb the herbs as they are drying.

For herbs with small leaves or those that shed leaves quickly when dried, like thyme, loosely secure a paper bag around the herb bundle to help you catch the leaves.

Oven drying is sometimes used for quick drying herbs, but it consumes quite a bit of energy to use this process, so I personally discourage relying on this method for long-term use. However, if you find yourself in a pinch, place the herbs on an oven safe drying rack with a baking pan underneath (to catch any leaves that fall off). Set the oven temperature to 120 degrees Fahrenheit.

Check the herbs every hour to test for dryness. When sufficiently dried, remove from oven and allow to cool prior to use.

Most spices can be easily dried, ideally with the assistance of a dehydrator.

As mentioned in the "Stocking Your Medicinal Kitchen" section, purchasing a dehydrator for drying medicinal garden produce is a smart option. There are plenty of energy-friendly models available for every budget.

Dehydrators can be used overnight, require little attention, have regulated temperatures, and have a low risk of burning. Air circulation in a dehydrator is at optimum levels, ensuring the plants all dry in the most efficient manner possible. As a bonus, they save space with their compact design. You won't need to spread out the herbs or spices over an entire room to dry them. With a multishelf dehydrator unit, you can easily dry a large batch of herbs in a fraction of the space.

Root spices can be sliced and dried easily with the use of a dehydrator. Garlic and onions are easy to dehydrate, as well, to be minced, ground, or powdered after.

It's best to cut open cayenne pepper and paprika and remove the seeds prior to dehydrating. Cayenne pepper seeds can be air dried separately if you enjoy using them in recipes.

For most herbs, you can remove the leaves prior to dehydrating and just lay them flat in the dehydrator. Optionally, for herbs like thyme, simply lay the stems with leaves intact in the dehydrator. Once the herbs are dried, remove stems and keep leaves whole. Keeping leaves whole will help them last a bit longer. You can crumble each leaf prior to using for cooking, bath water, or any other needs.

When fully dried, store in an airtight container in a cool, dark space like your pantry or a kitchen cabinet.

Optionally, grind herbs or spices, then store the ground herb or spice in an airtight container in a cool, dark space.

Label each container of dried herbs or spices and record, at a minimum, the name of the plant stored and the date preserved.

Dried herbs/spices will keep for around six months to a year. After that, the flavor begins to wane. Renew your supply at least once per year.

FRESH-BAKED TIP: When your dried herbs have expired, you can compost them or use them in creative ways such as:

- pouring them over hot coals in your fireplace to scent your home,
- adding them to hot coals in your barbecue grill outside to infuse flavor and scent to foods you're grilling, and
- tossing them onto hot coals in your outdoor fire-pit to add an aromatherapy component to your evening enjoyment.

To help keep the herbs dry and avoid molding, be sure to seal each container airtight initially and after each use.

Spices do not always age gracefully. Heat is one of the most common enemies. Do not store any fresh or dried herb or spice over a heated area. Ironically, the cabinet over the stove is where many people store their herbs and spices. This is not an ideal situation at all because, well, heat rises!

A cabinet next to the stove is not ideal either. A cabinet that is removed from the stove area by at least three feet is a better option. A pantry that is on the opposite side of the kitchen or separated from the kitchen is an even more ideal storage location. While you may need to take a few extra steps to gather herbs and spices prior to cooking or using them for your medicinal needs, it will be well worth the effort. You'll get a better return on longevity of freshness from your herbs and spices when they are stored properly.

 FRESH-BAKED TIP: For quick reference: one teaspoon of dried herbs equals approximately two to three teaspoons of fresh minced herbs.

WHAT'S THE BEST WAY TO PRESERVE HEMP AND CBD?

If you live in a state where you can grow your own cannabis plants, the best method for preservation of CBD flowers is to dry them, then vacuum seal. Store the vacuum-sealed package in a dark, dry space.

Freezing or refrigerating will degrade the plant, and light is an enemy, so do make sure they are kept in a dark area. If you store CBD flowers in your pantry and you frequently turn the light in the room on, place the vacuum bags in an opaque box with a lid to ensure they receive minimal light exposure.

The same is true for CBD oil and hempseed oil. It's best to limit light exposure and keep all cannabis plant-derived oils in a dark, dry space.

Hempseed oil requires refrigeration to extend viability. Outside of refrigeration, hempseed oil has a short shelf life, typically less than three months. You can extend the life of the product with refrigeration up to a year. It's best to keep it at the back of the refrigerator for optimal results, as the temperature will be the most consistent.

Hempseeds or hemp hearts should be stored in an airtight container in the refrigerator or the freezer. Shelf stable sealed bags of hempseeds purchased from your natural grocery store may be stored in your pantry, but once opened, be sure to place in an airtight container to store in the refrigerator or freezer. This will help preserve and extend the life of the product up to a year.

DRYING HERB SEEDS

Coriander, dill, celeriac, fennel, and mustard plants all produce excellent seeds for use in teas, pickling, and seasoning. Seeds should be harvested when fully formed before they are brittle or split. It's okay if some of the seeds are still slightly green when you harvest seeds for drying.

If seeds are split, the plant is getting ready to scatter seeds. Let nature take its course and you'll have a fresh crop of plants next season.

For drying the seeds, find a cool, dry spot with good air circulation and no direct sunlight. I like to set a table up in our guest bedroom and pull the shades closed. It's a good area to dry them in.

Lay out towels (or paper towels), then set up a mesh screen (or drying rack with a grid pattern) atop the towels. The towels will catch the seeds as they fall off and make it easier for you to gather them up after drying.

Lay stalks with seeds on the mesh screen and allow them to air dry. Typically, when you notice many of the seeds are falling off the stalk, they will be ready.

You can push a fingernail into the seeds to test if they are fully dry. If the seed gives under the pressure of your nail, they are not fully dry. The seeds should be very brittle to the touch and crush easily.

Once dried, remove any remaining seeds from the stalks by gently shaking them loose or brushing them off the stalks lightly with your fingertips.

Store dried seeds in an airtight container in a cool, dark space. Whole seeds are ideal for use with teas and pickling.

Alternatively, prior to storing, powder the dried seeds using an herb grinder or mortar and pestle.

In general, it's best to keep the dried seeds whole, rather than grinding them immediately, if you will be storing them for a long time. This helps preserve the freshness and flavor. Whole seeds can be stored for up to four years and you can grind the seeds as needed. Once ground, the storage life is shortened two years before flavor and freshness is lost.

DRYING CITRUS PEEL

Just like the fruits they house, citrus peels have vitamin C. The lovely sweet tang is terrific when used for flavoring in teas, olive oils, and recipes.

Their scent is also wonderful in homemade potpourri, cleaning solutions, and bath and beauty treatments. For aromatic purposes, you may want to consider adding a dwarf lemon or orange tree to your medicinal garden. You can easily grow them in large pots and reap a small crop each year.

If you're drying citrus peels from fruit you purchased at the grocer, be sure that you are purchasing organic fruits that have not been sprayed with chemicals. Even so, it's best to scrub the peels of all citrus fruits (before peeling or grating) to ensure you remove any dirt and potential toxins.

To dry, simply remove the peel from the fruit. Scrape off any remaining fruit.

Cut the peel into thin strips and lay flat on a drying rack in a cool, dry, dark space.

I prefer to use my dehydrator to dry fruit peels, as it works faster and reduces the chance of mold, but I've air-dried citrus peels many times, especially when I have a smaller batch.

When the peel is fully dried, it can be stored in an airtight container in a cool, dark space for use whole or ground into powder for recipes. When properly stored, dried peel can last up to two years, but you'll generally use up this delicious citrus goodness much quicker!

 FRESH-BAKED TIP: Re-create your favorite store spice blends using dried herbs and spices straight from your medicinal garden. Mix them up, label them, and store in the same manner as your dried herbs.

Try my favorite blends to help get you started:

SPICE MIX	INGREDIENTS
Italian Seasoning	1 tablespoon each of dried marjoram, thyme, rosemary, sage, oregano, and basil
Rosemary Mix	1 tablespoon each of dried rosemary, oregano, parsley, and thyme
Southwestern Seasoning	1 teaspoon ground cayenne pepper, 1 teaspoon ground cumin, 1 tablespoon onion powder, 1 tablespoon garlic powder
Asian Seasoning	1/2 teaspoon of ground chili pepper, plus 1 tablespoon each of garlic powder, ground ginger, ground orange peel, onion powder, and powdered chives
Chicken Seasoning	1 tablespoon each of garlic powder, onion powder, ground black pepper, parsley, paprika, and ground orange peel

SPICE MIX	INGREDIENTS (cont.)
Breakfast Blend	1 tablespoon each of ground turmeric, ground cinnamon, ground cardamom, ground ginger, and ground nutmeg
Allspice	1 tablespoon each of ground nutmeg, ground cinnamon, and ground cloves
Herbes de Provence	1 tablespoon each of dried thyme, basil, ground rosemary, marjoram, parsley, tarragon, and lavender flowers, plus 1/2 tablespoon of ground fennel
All-purpose Hemp Seasoning	1 tablespoon each of hemp protein powder, onion powder, and garlic powder, plus 1 teaspoon each of sea salt and ground black pepper
Steak Rub	1 tablespoon each of sea salt, ground black pepper, brown sugar, oregano, ground cumin, thyme, and sage
Coffee Steak Rub	Use same ingredients as Steak Rub but add 1 tablespoon of coarse coffee grounds
Barbecue Rub	1 tablespoon each of sea salt, brown sugar, mustard powder, paprika, and onion powder
All-purpose Rub	1 tablespoon each of sea salt, ground black pepper, garlic powder, onion powder, ground coriander, ground dill seed
French Fry Seasoning	1 tablespoon each of sea salt, ground black pepper, onion powder, ground celery seed, oregano, sage, garlic powder, paprika, and 1/2 tablespoon ground cumin
Bread Dip	1 tablespoon each of sea salt, minced garlic, parsley, onion powder, basil, ground rosemary, and sage.

ALCOHOL CURING YOUR MEDICINAL PLANTS

If you read my prior book, *Getting Laid: Everything You Need to Know About Raising Chickens, Gardening and Preserving*, you already know I'm a big fan of the lost art of alcohol preservation techniques. Once used prolifically, canning with alcohol is now pretty much relegated to moonshine cherries and bourbon vanilla extracts in the modern kitchen.

In the medicinal kitchen, alcohol extraction is a quick, easy way to make tinctures that's well worth exploring for the entry level herbalist. Some of the tinctures you create are also fun to use for artisan cocktails (more about that in Chapter 8)!

Alcohol tinctures have a long shelf life, generally up to two years, and can be used internally and externally. This method preserves all properties of the plant, including oils, flavor, and scent, in a quick and efficient manner.

It's important to note, if you are considering ingesting alcohol tinctures regularly, you will need to proceed with caution. Alcohol, even in small quantities, may have a negative effect if you are alcohol sensitive. It may also interfere with prescription medicines. It's always wise to consult your doctor and pharmacist prior to use.

To create alcohol herb tinctures, you will need:

- fresh herbs, cleaned and chopped
- clear vodka (or rum) 80-proof or higher
- 8-ounce mason jars
- fine mesh strainer (or cheesecloth)

Fill an eight-ounce mason jar halfway with fresh chopped herbs. Pour in vodka over herbs, filling jar completely. Seal the jar tightly.

Store jar in a cool, dry, dark space with good airflow (like a pantry shelf) for one month. Gently shake the jar regularly, once per day is ideal.

After the curing period of one month, open the jar and strain the mixture using a fine mesh strainer to separate the herbs from the alcohol. Return alcohol tincture to jar, discard herbs.

A typical dose of tincture is one teaspoon. It can be taken orally straight from the jar or mixed with your favorite beverage.

I enjoy using these tinctures to make medicinal herbal teas. When you use an alcohol tincture to make a hot tea, the alcohol generally dissipates, making this a preferred option for many medicinal gardeners. Simply add one teaspoon to eight ounces of boiling water to create the tea.

You can then add in ingredients like honey or a touch of maple syrup for sweetness, or lemon for an extra layer of tart flavor.

If you find that one teaspoon is just too strong for your taste, reduce the amount. I adore a strong peppermint or lemongrass tea, but am less enthusiastic about a strong sage tea, so I only add a half teaspoon of sage tincture when I brew a medicinal tea.

 FRESH-BAKED TIP: After straining the herbs from your alcohol herb tincture, instead of covering the jar with a lid, cover the opening with a piece of cheesecloth. Secure the cheesecloth with a rubber band or string to the top of the jar.

Leave the jar in a cool, dry, dark space for several weeks (or until alcohol completely evaporates). When the alcohol completely evaporates, the small amount left behind is essential oil that can be used in DIY bath and beauty products or to scent potpourri and homemade air fresheners.

PICKLING YOUR MEDICINAL PLANTS

Herbs like dill and coriander are wildly popular for pickling, as they add complexity and desirable flavor attributes to pickled foods. Pickled spices like onions, ginger, and paprika add a bit of zing and an element of fun to salads, sandwiches, and charcuterie boards.

It's perhaps not the best method of preserving your medicinal garden, but certainly a great way to use extra herbs and spices for variation, allowing you to enjoy them in a new way. Fermented foods also contain healthy bacteria, which may help your digestive system.

There are four primary types of vinegar available for use in pickling:

- white distilled vinegar made from alcohol
- cider vinegar made from apples
- wine vinegar made from grape wine
- brown rice vinegar distilled from brown rice sake.

Each has its own unique flavor profile.

You'll find a wealth of pickling recipes with a quick search on the internet, including my tried and true Garlic Dill Pickle recipe (www.ruralmom.com/2014/08/garlic-dill-pickles-canning-recipe-tips.html). My favorite medicinal garden pickling recipe is pickled shallots. It's a fantastic way to enjoy the rich goodness of this spice and a lovely ingredient to help liven up your daily recipes.

BARB'S QUICK PICKELED SHALLOTS

Yield: six 4-ounce jars or three 8-ounce jars

Ingredients:
3 cups brown rice vinegar
1/2 cup sugar
3 cups of shallots

In a small saucepan over a medium heat, add vinegar and sugar. Stir regularly until sugar is fully dissolved. Remove from heat and allow to cool.

Trim the tops of shallots, remove outer dry skin, and clean shallots. Fill mason jar with shallots.

Pour vinegar over shallots, filling jar to rim. Seal jar and refrigerate for one week. After one week, use and enjoy!

Jars may be stored in the refrigerator for up to one year.

VINEGAR CURING YOUR MEDICINAL PLANTS

Vinegar isn't just a great ingredient to use for pickling your medicinal garden produce, it's a fantastic medium to use for creating marinades, salad dressings, drinks, and tinctures.

Herb-infused vinegar tinctures are created using the same method as alcohol herb tinctures. The only difference is that you warm the vinegar (simply warm, not boil) prior to pouring it over the herbs. This helps speed up the infusion process.

Vinegar tinctures can be used daily by the spoonful. Medicinal garden-infused vinegars are also a low-calorie way to add intense flavor to your beverages. They can be added to eight ounces of soda water to create a refreshing drink or added to hot water to make a medicinal tea. Add a squeeze of lemon, orange, lime, or grapefruit juice and/or a tiny bit of stevia or organic sugar to sweeten things up.

My all-time favorite is to add lemon verbena-infused vinegar to soda water with a little bit of lime, which tastes just like it sounds—a lemon-lime soda. I also love to add a bit of rosemary-infused vinegar and a squeeze of lemon to iced black tea as a summer refresher.

For using infused vinegars to create custom marinades and dressings, refer to the "Creating Medicinal Plant-Infused Food-Grade Oils" section in this chapter.

 FRESH-BAKED TIP: You can use your multicooker to infuse vinegar!

Respecting the traditions of the past is an important aspect of the medicinal herbalist's life. There's a reason methods like brewing medicinal teas and pickling with herbs have stood the test of time: they work.

Over the years, equipment like electric tea kettles, kitchen blenders, and electric food dehydrators have certainly enhanced and improved our ability to preserve and utilize medicinal plants more efficiently. A kitchen tool that's currently a culinary darling for many home chefs is the multicooker. This clever gadget has the ability to remarkably speed up your medicinal garden vinegar infusions.

Apple cider vinegar is the ideal choice when using a multicooker for an herb-vinegar infusion. Use one cup of fresh herbs per two cups of vinegar.

Simply add the herbs and vinegar to your multicooker. Following the manufacturer's directions for your multicooker, pressure cook for thirty minutes.

Again, following the manufacturer's instructions, allow the multicooker to release pressure and cool down. When venting and resting period is complete, open the multicooker. Allow liquid to completely cool.

Pour vinegar and herbs into eight-ounce mason jars. Seal and store in a cool, dry, dark spot for twenty-four hours. After twenty-four hours, strain plant materials from vinegar and discard the herbs.

As you can see, this takes the process of infusing vinegar from one month to two days!

There's a lot to be said for using the tried-and-true old methods of preservation, but there's plenty of benefits to using our modern conveniences to speed things up from time to time.

CREATING MEDICINAL PLANT-INFUSED FOOD-GRADE OILS

Preserving medicinal herbs and spices with food-grade oils is not a long-term storage solution, as they degrade quickly, and the oils have a short shelf life to begin with. Infused oils should be used within one week of infusing.

Because of this, it's a good choice to use your medicinal herbs for salad dressings, bread dips, marinades, and for finishing recipes. Drizzling basil-infused olive oil over pan-fried chicken or garlic-infused oil over baked zucchini prior to serving is totally delicious.

Since they have a short shelf life, it's best not to make a large batch and to plan to use infused oils within one week.

The best oils to use are avocado oil, sunflower oil, and olive oil.

To infuse oil with medicinal garden plants, you will need one-third cup fresh herbs or spices per two cups of oil, as well as clean glass jars with tight seals. A mason jar works well, or you can use a specialty glass jar designed for housing oils. I like to save my empty olive oil jars, clean them, and repurpose them for use.

To create medicinal plant-infused oil, clean and dry herbs or spices (like sliced ginger root or peeled garlic). Add medicinal plants to jar. Fill remainder of jar with oil.

As you are filling the jar, swirl it gently to help coat the herbs/spices with oil.

Seal jar tightly and store in a cool, dark, dry space for one week.

After one week, use a fine mesh strainer to strain medicinal plant matter from the oil into another vessel. Dispose of plant matter and return oil to jar. Use oil immediately or reseal and store in refrigerator for later use.

Shelf life will vary depending upon the oil used. When using oils, always look for signs of spoilage. If at any time you notice the oil is cloudy or has an unexpected foul odor, discard the oil properly and do not consume. Consult the Food Safety Standards at https://www.foodsafety.gov for the most up-to-date information.

To create marinades and salad dressings, mix two-thirds cup of herb-infused oil with one-third cup of vinegar (of choice). This produces a simple oil and vinegar dressing.

It's incredibly fun (and rewarding to your taste buds) to pair herb-infused oils with herb-infused vinegars for marinades and dressings.

Some of my favorite combinations include:

- garlic oil + basil vinegar
- rosemary oil + sage vinegar
- chamomile oil + lemon verbena vinegar
- lemongrass oil + thyme vinegar

Jazz up your salad dressings by adding in one tablespoon of fresh chopped herbs, one-half teaspoon of dill honey mustard (recipe in Chapter 7), and a pinch of sea salt and pepper.

FRESH-BAKED TIP: A rosemary olive oil hair mask is a wonderful beauty treatment to try. A scalp soother and hair moisturizer, this DIY beauty fix can reduce dandruff and leave your locks looking lush.

To use, warm a cup of rosemary-infused olive oil in the microwave for ten seconds (or until warm to the touch). If you overheat the oil, allow it to cool down. You just want it warm, not too hot, or it could potentially burn your scalp.

Massage oil into hair and leave in for twenty minutes. After twenty minutes has passed, rinse hair thoroughly, towel hair gently, and allow hair to air dry. Then wash and condition your hair as you normally would.

I sometimes use this treatment at night, then shower in the morning with my normal shampoo routine.

PRODUCING THERAPEUTIC ESSENTIAL OILS FROM YOUR MEDICINAL PLANTS

Essential oils are concentrated extracts that are generally used as aromatics. They capture the plant's flavor and scent and are often used in aromatherapy, household cleaners, or bath and skin-care products.

Therapeutic essential oils are not designed for consumption. They are meant to be used in small doses in aromatherapy and DIY projects, as they are quite potent.

The scents of essential oils are mood enhancers. Lemon essential oil can energize your senses and evoke feelings of happiness. A dab of peppermint essential oil on your temples may help relieve headache pain.

I'm a huge fan of using essential oils to freshen my home. You can use them in a diffuser, add a few drops to your potpourri, and even create homemade air fresheners.

FRESH-BAKED TIP: Use this quick and easy recipe to create a lovely homemade air freshening spray.

For this recipe, you'll need:

- 16 ounces clean spray bottle (a great opportunity to recycle old spray bottles)
- purified or distilled water (at room temperature)
- the essential oil (or oils) of your choice.

I love to use grapefruit essential oil in the kitchen, it's such a bright scent. Peppermint essential oil is a holiday favorite, plus a great pick-me-up energizing scent. Lavender essential oil has a nice soothing scent, perfect for creating a restful atmosphere in the evening.

You can also try combining scents for your own custom creation, like lavender and vanilla or lemon and rosemary.

To create the air freshener, fill the spray bottle with water, leaving approximately a one-inch headspace at the top.

Next, use eight to ten drops of your favorite essential oils (adjust amount to your liking) and shake for thirty seconds.

Spritz a little of your homemade air freshener where needed and enjoy the lovely toxin-free scent!

Be sure to shake the bottle before each use for the best results.

If you're in a pinch and don't have a water purifier in your home or distilled water on hand, simply make a small batch of air freshener. Use one drop of essential oil for every two ounces of water.

Untreated water can have impurities that you may not wish to spray around your home, like fluoride, chlorine, and salts, so it's generally better to avoid using water that hasn't been purified first.

Essential oils can be produced at home, but it does take mass quantities of herbs to produce them.

For example: You will need around three pounds of lavender flowers to make one average size jar (15 ml) of lavender essential oil.

If you have a small garden, it's daunting to attempt to grow and make all the essential oils you need for the year. It's much easier and more practical to purchase essentials oils for use in your health and beauty regimens from a local distributor.

When purchasing essential oils always:

1. Seek out quality manufacturers. Look for chemical-free therapeutic-grade products produced through distillation or mechanical cold processing.
2. Pay close attention to the ingredients. The essential oil should be pure. It shouldn't have any additives.

If you want to give making essential oils at home a whirl, using a slow cooker is a quick and relatively easy way to begin.

If you think you will be making essential oils regularly and long term, you'll want to research further and invest in advanced equipment like a copper still.

SLOW COOKER ESSENTIAL OILS

Items you will need for making essential oils with your slow cooker are:

- 6-quart slow cooker with removable pot (if your slow cooker doesn't have a removable pot, you'll also need a 6-quart casserole dish with a lid)
- concave rubber spatula for skimming oils off water (a soup spoon also works well)
- 4-ounce mason jar (*or smaller*)
- 1 gallon of distilled water
- 4 cups of fresh chopped herbs

Note: If you are using a slow cooker with a capacity larger than six quarts, you may want to increase the amount of your water and herbs. If you are using one smaller than six quarts, decrease the ingredients accordingly.

To make slow-cooker essential oils, add chopped herbs to the slow cooker. The herbs should ideally fill the slow cooker about halfway full.

Add water to the slow cooker to cover herbs. Do not fill the slow cooker more than three-fourths of the way full.

Cover slow cooker. Heat on high for one hour. After one hour, reduce heat to low and simmer for four hours.

When herbs are finished simmering, remove pot from slow cooker with lid attached and place on a trivet to cool. Allow slow-cooker pot to cool down for one hour. Do not remove lid during this time.

Place slow-cooker pot, with lid cover still on, into the refrigerator. Chill for twenty-four hours.

Alternatively, if your slow cooker does not have a detachable pot—after slow cooker has finished cooking, allow slow cooker to cool down for one hour. Do not remove lid during this time. After one hour, transfer slow-cooker ingredients into a six-quart casserole dish. Use a spatula to scrape sides and inside of the lid of the slow cooker to transfer all liquid and plant materials into the casserole dish. Seal casserole dish with its lid and place into the refrigerator. Chill for twenty-four hours.

After twenty-four hours, remove slow cooker from refrigerator. There will be a thin film of oil at the top of the water (and often on the inside of the lid). Working quickly, skim oil from the top of the water and lid and transfer into a mason jar.

Viola! You now have a small batch of essential oils!

Seal the jar and store in a cool, dark spot. Use for bath and beauty products, DIY bug sprays, or aromatherapy, as needed.

It is generally a lot quicker and easier to purchase essentials oils, but if you have an excess of lavender or peppermint on hand, it can be a fun way to capture some therapeutic scents for your bath rituals or homemade goodies like potpourri.

Adding Hemp, CBD, and Medicinal Plants to Your Recipes

CBD, hemp, and medicinal gardening produce are all terrific diet supplements, and can be conveniently incorporated into your favorite cuisines.

Hempseeds add texture and a delightful nutty flavor. Incorporating CBD isolate powder or full-spectrum CBD oil into some of your favorite recipes is a fun, easy way to ingest your daily dose. Herbs and spices liven up every dish, turning an ordinary meal into a culinary adventure for your taste buds.

All also add an extra element of self-care and healthful attributes to each meal.

Most herbs and spices will remain fresh for several days. Others, up to several weeks with proper storage. To keep them viable longer, turn to Chapter 6 for long-term storage solutions.

Likely, you already have your favorite recipes and ideas in mind for all your herbs and spices, but if you're wondering what exactly to pair your tarragon up with, here's a handy idea chart for your reference. These are all combinations that I've learned work well from my forty-plus years of home cooking and fifteen-plus years of professional recipe development.

There's not really a 100 percent definitive guide to herb/spice and food pairings, as it's subjective to personal taste. Chefs and food manufacturers around the world continue to experiment with new flavor combinations. This guide is a starting point—certainly use your own creativity in the kitchen and let your taste buds be the ultimate guide!

COMMON FOOD PAIRINGS FOR HERBS AND SPICES

HERB/SPICE	PAIRS WELL WITH
Ashwagandha	broccoli, carrots, cauliflower, celeriac, eggplant, green beans, peas, potatoes, peppers, spinach
Basil/Holy Basil	asparagus, beef, beets, cheese, chicken, eggs, fish, peas, salad, squash, tomatoes, turkey
Bay Leaf	chicken, tomato sauce, soup, stews, venison
Cardamom	apples, baked goods, beans, Indian cuisine, orange, pears
Cayenne Pepper	beef, chicken, chocolate, green beans, lime, mushrooms, potatoes, spinach and greens, tomatoes, turkey, zucchini
Celeriac	beef, chicken salad, coriander, fennel, fish, paprika, potato salad, salads
Chamomile	desserts, fish, salads, shellfish
Chives	beets, broccoli, cheese, corn, cucumbers, eggs, fish, green beans, potatoes, radishes, spinach, tomatoes, zucchini
Cilantro/Coriander	artichoke, avocado, beef, beets, carrots, cauliflower, celeriac, chicken, corn, fish, lamb, lemon, lime, mushrooms, orange, peppers, pork, potatoes, salsa, tomatoes
Cinnamon	apple, bananas, chicken, desserts, pears, pumpkin, sweet fish, sweet potatoes
Clove	beef, beets, desserts, orange, pork, pumpkin, squash, sweet potatoes
Cumin	beans, beets, cauliflower, chicken, eggplant, lamb, mushrooms, potatoes, pumpkin, tomatoes, turkey

HERB/SPICE	PAIRS WELL WITH (cont.)
Dill	asparagus, beans, beets, cabbage, carrots, chicken, corn, cucumber, egg salad, fish, green beans, lamb, peas, pickled vegetables, potatoes, radish, sour cream, spinach, tomatoes
Edible Flowers	all-purpose garnish, desserts, salads, soups
Fennel	beef, beets, celeriac, fish, pork, salads, tomatoes
Garlic	other than desserts, there are plenty of recipes that utilize the merits of garlic. It pairs with every vegetable and meat brilliantly
Ginger	apples, beets, broccoli, cauliflower, chocolate, eggplant, fish, mushrooms, pears, pineapple, pork, pumpkin
Ginseng	all meats and most vegetables, ginseng is great to add to stir-fry
Lavender	apples, berries, desserts, lamb, peaches, oranges
Lemon Balm	chicken, desserts, fish, salads, and use as a grated lemon peel substitute for any recipe
Lemongrass	beef, chicken, coconut, fish, pork, shellfish
Lemon Verbena	chicken, chocolate, desserts, fruits, fish, pork
Marjoram	asparagus, beef, celeriac, chicken, fish, peas, pork, soups, stuffing, zucchini
Mint	fruits, cauliflower, chocolate, cucumber, desserts, eggplant, fish, lamb, peas, pork, potatoes, radish, salads
Mustard	asparagus, beef, Brussels sprouts, chicken, cucumber, eggs, fish, green beans, pork, potatoes
Nutmeg	asparagus, beets, broccoli, cheese, chicken, cucumber, eggs, fish, pickles, salads, shellfish, tomatoes

HERB/SPICE	PAIRS WELL WITH (cont.)
Onion/Shallot	beef, chicken, corn, fish, game meats, green beans, peas, pork, soups, stews, tomatoes, zucchini
Oregano	artichokes, asparagus, beef, broccoli, chicken, eggplant, fish, green beans, pork, potatoes, tomatoes, turkey, zucchini
Paprika	artichoke, cauliflower, celeriac, chicken, corn, eggs, fish, potatoes, pumpkin, squash, sweet potatoes, tomatoes, turkey
Parsley	Everything! Use as a fresh garnish or finishing ingredient for any meal.
Rosemary	apricots, asparagus, beans, beef, broccoli, Brussels sprouts, cauliflower, chicken, corn, eggs, fish, green beans, lamb, peppers, pork, potatoes, pumpkin, soups, stews, stuffing, turkey
Saffron	beans, chicken, corn, eggs, fish, lamb, pork, shellfish, turkey
Sage	beans, beef, beets, chicken, fish, peas, pork, potatoes, pumpkin, sausage, stuffing, sweet potatoes, turkey, venison
Tarragon	asparagus, beets, broccoli, cheese, chicken, cucumber, eggs, fish, pickles, salads, shellfish, tomatoes
Thyme	beans, beef, beets, broccoli, cauliflower, celeriac, cheese, chicken, corn, eggs, fish, green beans, mushrooms, pork, potatoes, pumpkin, salads, stews, stuffing, sweet potatoes, turkey
Turmeric	beans, chicken, curries, eggplant, fish, lamb, spinach and other greens, also used as a saffron substitute.

FRESH-BAKED TIP: Thyme is truly a versatile herb that pairs well with so many foods. Packed with vitamin C, antioxidants, and a mood-boosting scent, it's also revered for its potential health benefits.

If you aren't feeling well, my favorite medicinal garden comfort food—thyme soup—may help perk you up.

MEDICINAL GARDEN THYME SOUP

Yield: Serves 2-4

Ingredients:

4 cups vegetable stock
1 onion, diced
1 cup celeriac, diced
2 tablespoons fresh thyme leaves,
  chopped
1 clove garlic, diced
2 tablespoons extra-virgin olive
  oil
sea salt and pepper

In a medium saucepan, over a medium heat, warm olive oil. Add onion and celeriac. Sauté for five minutes (or until soft and translucent). Add garlic, sauté for one minute.

Add vegetable stock and thyme. Reduce heat to medium-low and simmer for thirty minutes, stirring occasionally.

Remove from heat, add salt and pepper, to taste. Serve with a side of bread and enjoy!

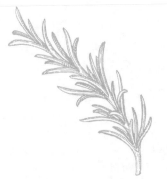

RECIPE MEASUREMENT EQUIVALENCY CHEAT SHEET

Fresh herbs, ground spices, CBD oil, hempseeds—they all have various methods of measurement. When you're dealing with your favorite recipes, you often need to find the equivalents quickly.

Copy this chart and tape it to the inside of your spice cabinet, or laminate and glue it on a magnet to secure to your refrigerator for quick reference.*

CUP	TBSP	TSP	FLUID OUNCE	ML
1 cup	16 tbsp.	48 tsp.	8 oz.	237 ml
3/4 cup	12 tbsp.	36 tsp.	6 oz.	177 ml
2/3 cup	11 tbsp.	32 tsp.	5 oz.	158 ml
1/2 cup	8 tbsp.	24 tsp.	4 oz.	118 ml
1/3 cup	5 tbsp.	16 tsp.	3 oz.	79 ml
1/4 cup	4 tbsp.	12 tsp.	2 oz.	59 ml
1/8 cup	2 tbsp.	6 tsp.	1 oz.	30 ml
1/16 cup	1 tbsp.	3 tsp.	.5 oz.	15 ml

*Measurements are rounded to closest equivalent.

USING CBD IN A RECIPE?

Always be mindful of dose. Don't use CBD oil or powder as an ingredient substitute.

For example: Mint flavored CBD oils have a refreshing element in taste. You think it will be fun to add it to your hummus recipe.

Let's say your hummus recipe that makes four servings calls for one tablespoon of extra-virgin olive oil to top it off. You ideally want 20 mg of CBD oil per portion.

Swapping 15 ml (the equivalent of one ttablespoon) of CBD oil for the extra-virgin olive oil is not a good idea. If your 15 ml bottle of CBD oil contains 600 mg of CBD, you would essentially add 600 mg of CBD, resulting in 150 mg of CBD per portion.

That would be adding over seven times the amount of CBD you wanted in each portion. Way more than you need!

The ideal route to follow is to create your hummus recipe and portion it into four servings. Then, drizzle your olive oil equally onto each portion. Lastly, top one portion of hummus off with your normal 20 mg dose (typically 1 ml) of CBD oil directly prior to consuming. Store the remaining portions of hummus and again, directly prior to consuming, top off with your desired dose of CBD oil.

This way your dose will be accurate, the potency fresh, and the hint of flavor from the CBD oil will not be overpowering.

SHOULD YOU USE CBD OIL IN YOUR RECIPES?

CBD oil can be used in your recipes when you're looking for an occasional change in your preferred supplement delivery method. If you just aren't a big fan of the taste and texture of sublingual tinctures, this could be a great option for you.

When you use CBD in an edible format, do keep in mind that your absorption rate may vary. As you'll be ingesting CBD with various foods that digest at various rates, the rate of absorption in your body may fluctuate.

CBD-infused edibles are still a speculative and relatively uncharted territory. When you mix your CBD oil with any food substance, it may decrease the effect, shorten or lengthen the effect period, and/or add an undesirable earthy hemp flavor to your foods.

On the flipside, CBD-infused snacks can provide you with an alternative delivery system that's portable and easy to incorporate into your daily lifestyle. This is beneficial especially when you're on the go or you wish to be more discreet with dosing.

FRESH-BAKED TIP: If you don't like the flavor of straight CBD oil (it can be overpowering), try mixing your next dose with a teaspoon of almond butter or any other nut butter you prefer. Research shows that taking CBD with fatty foods (like nut butters) can also increase absorption.[36]

Another great option is to make a CBD Peppermint Cocoa Bomb. This is my favorite quick recipe for a delicious snack CBD edible. It's great for packing in your lunchbox as a midday treat or enjoying at the end of the day along with a cup of warm medicinal tea.

If you're familiar with the Keto diet or other popular diets, this recipe may look familiar. This style of treat, often referred to as a "fat bomb," is very popular. I've updated this style of treat with an infusion of CBD and a twist of peppermint-infused honey.

Not a fan of peppermint? No worries! You can use regular honey or any other herb-infused honey you prefer. (See the "Herb-Infused Honey" section later in this chapter for directions on using your medicinal herbs to create flavorful honey infusions.)

To make my CBD Peppermint Cocoa Bombs, you will need:

- 1/2 cup almond butter
- 1/2 cup coconut oil
- 1/2 cup cocoa powder
- 1 teaspoon of peppermint-infused honey
- 2 ml of CBD oil (to equal desired dose*)
- silicone ice-cube tray

*To determine your desired dose of CBD per Peppermint Cocoa Bomb, divide your 2 ml CBD dose by ten servings (the number of cocoa bombs this recipe creates).

For example: If each milliliter of CBD oil contains 30 mg of CBD, then 2 ml will contain 60 mg of CBD. Therefore, 60 ml divided by ten servings equals 6 mg of CBD per cocoa bomb. If you want a higher dose per serving, you will need to choose a CBD oil containing a higher milligram dose of CBD per milliliter. Ideally, do not exceed 2 ml of CBD oil total for this recipe, as it can alter the outcome.

To make: in a small nonstick saucepan, over a low heat, add the coconut oil. Heat until fully melted.

Add the cocoa powder. Whisk until fully incorporated and smooth.

Add almond butter. Whisk until fully incorporated and smooth.

Remove from heat.

Add honey and CBD oil. Whisk until fully incorporated and smooth.

Divide liquid evenly into ten individual ice-cube tray compartments.

Refrigerate tray for twenty-four hours. Remove tray from refrigerator and pop out Peppermint Cocoa Bombs. Place cocoa bombs in an airtight container in a single layer (or use wax paper to separate multiple layers in container). Store in refrigerator for up to two weeks.

Another point to take into consideration is that high temperatures used in cooking may degrade active compounds in cannabis.

There are some specialty CBD-infused cooking oils now available for use that help address this concern. Again, use your discretion when purchasing and always investigate the source and quality. Do be very cautious with CBD-infused products available on the market. Even fewer regulations exist for CBD edibles than tinctures, as this delivery method has not been approved by the FDA. Remember that you should consult a doctor or other health care professional before incorporating CBD into your food or beverages, and you should only purchase legal products.

When the FDA approved Epidiolex, the drug containing CBD used for treating epilepsy, the regulation waters got very murky. If CBD falls under a drug classification, then it is subject to our current drug laws, under which pharmaceutical drugs are not permitted to be added to foods.

In the same way you do not see Ibuprofen-infused yogurt or antihistamine pickles on grocery shelves, it's not yet legal for companies to market CBD by adding it to a food or labeling it as a dietary supplement, either.

There is legislative action underway, including Bill H.R. 5587[37] and Bill H.R. 8179,[38] to potentially extend the use of FDA-regulated cannabis plant materials to be used as dietary supplement additives in food and beverages. As regulations do change, you can find the most current information at fda.gov in the "Consumer Updates" section.

Despite the questions of legality, consumers still have access to CBD edibles and beverages via restaurants and food producers. As the regulations are still in question and the FDA has yet to fully weigh in, it has created sort of a murky sea where companies are testing the waters and the government has yet to step in and patrol them.

This is why you see items like CBD-infused coffee, water, ice cream, popcorn, simple syrups, chocolate truffles, caramels, cookies, and lollipops gaining in popularity. Some companies skirt around the issue by calling their products "full-spectrum hemp" and only indicating elsewhere on the label, such as in the list of ingredients, that the product contains cannabinoids like CBD.

Eventually we will see more regulatory measures in place. Currently, there's extraordinarily little research or scientific data to back up any claim that these products are an effective way to ingest CBD.

As with any other CBD product, do your research if you're considering purchase. Apply everything you learned in Chapters 2 and 3 when shopping for any product containing CBD.

When you're tempted to purchase CBD-infused cake pops or caramel corn, always listen to your body, as well. Those gourmet goodies you just shelled out $10–$20 apiece for may taste wonderful, but are they helping you in the same way your normal CBD oil dose is? Are they effective in treating your specific health concerns?

One of the reasons edibles are popular to manufacture is that companies can overinflate prices on CBD-infused products because they are trendy. Save yourself some money and splurge on regular gourmet caramel corn instead, and enjoy a handful after you take your CBD oil dose each day.

BEST METHODS FOR USING CBD IN RECIPES

If you decide you'd like to try cooking with CBD, the easiest recipes to start with are drinks and baked goods. (We'll be covering beverages in-depth in the next chapter.)

Rachel King, founder and chief development officer of Kaneh Co. (kanehedibles.

com), an elevated cannabis edibles brand, enjoys educating people to ensure they have a quality experience when consuming edibles. With her background as a pastry chef, she's well in tune with the sweeter side of the food spectrum and told me she's not surprised to find that gummies are one of the most popular edibles on the market.

"Chocolate, spices, mango, lemon, and most fat-based recipes enhance the experience of consuming cannabis," says King. "An easy way to begin is to buy a CBD-infused chocolate bar and make s'mores with it. Or purchase prepackaged cookies infused with CBD and make ice cream sandwiches with them."

King recommends home chefs start by adding CBD oil tinctures to their personal recipes at home. This is a good way to start gradually introducing CBD to your cooking routine.

To add CBD oil to your baking recipes, you'll generally want to first mix it with your wet ingredients. The reason is that when you mix your ingredients for your baked goods, such as a muffin, mixing all your wet ingredients plus your CBD oil directly prior to adding them to your dry ingredients helps ensure a more even and consistent distribution of CBD oil throughout the entire batch.

You'll also need to decide up front how many milligrams of CBD you'd ideally like in each portion. Once you determine the amount you would like to have in each portion, for example a 10 mg dose of CBD per muffin, you will need to multiply that by the number of portions in the recipe.

Note: To help you figure out how many milliliters of CBD oil to include in the recipe, based on the concentration of CBD in your CBD oil product, use the chart from Chapter 2.

Additional adjustments may also need to be made. When using CBD oil in a recipe, you're adding extra liquid to the recipe, which can affect the outcome. If you add 15 ml of CBD oil to a cake recipe, that's the equivalent of 1/16 of a cup or one tablespoon. To compensate, you may want to consider reducing one of the other liquid ingredients in the recipe, such as vegetable oil, milk, cream, or water, by one tablespoon.

This sounds complicated, and it may take a few minutes the first time you bake with CBD oil to ensure you have the right proportions, but once you go through the process, it will be very easy to follow the steps for all future recipes. I've included an illustration to help you visualize how this process works.

Baking with CBD Sample

Desired dose equals 10 milligrams of CBD per brownie. The typical brownie recipe yields 12 brownies. You will need a total of 120 milligrams of CBD for your recipe.

10 mg CBD oil per brownie x 12 brownies = 120 mg of CBD oil

Your CBD oil tincture bottle contains 30 ml of CBD oil with 150 milligrams of CBD in total. Each 1 ml serving contains 5 milligrams of CBD. You will need 24 ml of CBD oil for your recipe.

120 mg CBD / 5 mg = 24 ml doses = approx. 5 teaspoons

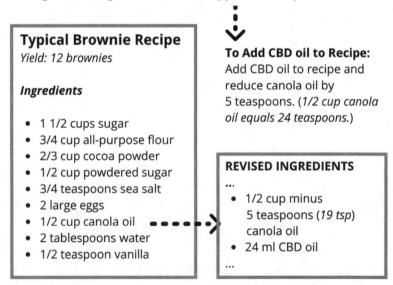

Typical Brownie Recipe
Yield: 12 brownies

Ingredients

- 1 1/2 cups sugar
- 3/4 cup all-purpose flour
- 2/3 cup cocoa powder
- 1/2 cup powdered sugar
- 3/4 teaspoons sea salt
- 2 large eggs
- 1/2 cup canola oil
- 2 tablespoons water
- 1/2 teaspoon vanilla

To Add CBD oil to Recipe:
Add CBD oil to recipe and reduce canola oil by 5 teaspoons. (*1/2 cup canola oil equals 24 teaspoons.*)

REVISED INGREDIENTS
...
- 1/2 cup minus 5 teaspoons (*19 tsp*) canola oil
- 24 ml CBD oil
...

Not all recipes will require a conversion. If you're using a very small amount of CBD, such as 1 or 2 ml, it will have little effect on a recipe. In such cases, just add the CBD oil when you add the other wet ingredients and continue with your recipe instructions per usual.

Some baked goods, like brownies, may be enhanced by added moisture. If you like ooey-gooey brownies and cookies, feel free to experiment by adding in the CBD oil without making a recipe adjustment. You may find it gives you an even more moist brownie than you previously thought possible.

In the beginning, however, it's best to make the modifications to ensure the success of your recipe. CBD oil is expensive, and it can be a costly mistake if your experiment flops. Once you're comfortable your recipe is turning out well, you can play around with the ingredients a little more until you find the 100 percent ideal recipe mix for you.

When sautéing or frying, CBD oil does not stand up to high heat like other cooking oils. Scientific research currently shows the boiling point of CBD as being between 320 and 356 degrees Fahrenheit.[39] When grilling, frying, or cooking with high temperatures, it is likely to destroy the potency, as the CBD will begin to degrade and/or evaporate. In these instances, it's best to incorporate CBD as a finishing ingredient, after you remove them from the heat source.

King suggests gradually adding CBD oil near the end of a recipe, stirring it into sauces before pouring them over a dish, or drizzling a bit of oil over plated foods directly prior to serving. Her additional tips include measuring the tincture ahead of making the recipe and always selecting top-notch ingredients.

"Whether you are infusing CBD oil, making things like cannabutter, or purchasing CBD-infused olive oil from a dispensary, it's important to make sure you have proper testing results to review," says King. "If you are a home grower, take it to a lab. You need to understand how much CBD or THC is in each dose to be sure you don't have a bad experience by adding too much to a recipe."

If you live in a state where CBD flowers are available for purchase or you have the ability to grow CBD-rich cannabis plants in your medicinal garden, a great option is to create your own CBD-infused butter for use in recipes.

Infusing the butter with CBD will help to distribute it more evenly in the recipe.

This is a popular technique commonly referred to as creating "cannabutter." You can find plenty of recipes and tutorials for creating a batch with a quick Google search. You'll even find specialty appliances for sale specifically designed to make cannabutter.

Cannabutter can be used in any recipe that already calls for butter. It may, however, change the flavor profile of the recipe. All cannabis plants have a strong flavor and scent that will come through in nearly every recipe. I'm not a huge fan of cooking with cannabis plants, and sometimes hempseed oils, for this reason.

While researching for this chapter, I had the chance to interview health and wellness expert Chef Crystal Blanchette (chefcrystalzworld.com) who regularly works with athletes, entertainers, and other clients who are interested in improving body wellness. First and foremost, she recommends slowly introducing CBD into your diet where it is most comfortable to help avoid having issues with flavor profiles.

"A lot of people love initially pairing alcohol with CBD," says Chef Blanchette. "Red wine is the way to go, as it drowns out the taste or bitterness."

Another way to get around the flavor of the cannabis plant is to use a CBD isolate powder when baking. You can mix the powder in with your wet ingredients before adding your dry ingredients to help distribute the CBD throughout the recipe.

As with using a CBD oil tincture, you will want to decide how much CBD isolate powder you will need for your recipe to ensure you have the proper amount per portion.

Unlike using a CBD oil tincture, you will not need to modify the recipe ingredients in any way, as the powder amount will be miniscule and should not affect the recipe outcome.

Alternatively, you can use CBD isolate powder to make your own CBD-infused oil for a recipe. The easiest way to do this is to warm the oil slightly, then mix in the CBD isolate powder until it is fully incorporated. Allow the oil to return to room temperature, then proceed with mixing your recipe ingredients per normal.

The drawback to using a CBD isolate powder, however, is that it is an isolate. If you use CBD isolate, you'll be missing all the other elements of the plant, including other plant compounds, oils, and terpenes contained in full-spectrum or broad-spectrum CBD oil.

"Once you are comfortable consuming CBD edibles, really play around with CBD oils and honeys," suggests Chef Blanchette. "Put CBD oil in spaghetti sauce or drizzle a few drops in your soup. It's a great way to trick your mind into a comfortable space when you are merely adding a small element to foods you already love."

Micro-dosing is a technique Chef Blanchette supports, as well. "Micro-dosing," in this context, refers to a trendy term that means administering half-doses or low doses of a CBD product. A micro-dose may even be as low as 10 percent of the suggested product dose.

"You never know how your body will react, and micro-dosing can be a deciding factor in whether you have a good or bad experience adding CBD to your mealtime," says Chef Blanchette. "Spend time to accurately measure your amounts. You can always take the full dose, but it's better to initially take half with your meal and then add in more later."

Lastly, Chef Blanchette suggests testing out various forms in cooking until you find something you enjoy. CBD salts, powders, oils, and specialty syrup products are all available, or will be available soon for home consumer use.

No doubt, you'll soon see CBD-infused butter, flour, and other cooking ingredients for sale at local markets. You know the drill by now—yup, do your due diligence and be sure to research the products thoroughly before purchasing.

 FRESH-BAKED TIP: Did you know you can make your own CBD-infused gummies? It's quite easy and, as a bonus, you can control the natural flavorings. You can even use flavoring straight from your medicinal garden, like chamomile, lavender, thyme, and lemongrass. Mint grapefruit gummies are my favorite flavor combo.

To make CBD-infused gummies you'll need small gummy molds. These are available for purchase online and at your local craft stores.

You first need to decide how many milligrams of CBD you want each gummy to have. My recipe makes about one hundred small bear-shaped gummies. Reasonably, you can add 15 ml of CBD oil to the recipe.

If your 15 ml bottle of CBD contains 500 mg of CBD, there will be approximately 5 mg of CBD in each gummy. You may also use a CBD isolate powder, instead of CBD oil, if preferred.

Keep in mind, as you are not working in a controlled lab with exact scientific measurements, some of the gummy candies may wind up with a higher concentration of CBD oil than others.

For my mint grapefruit recipe, you will need:

- 1/2 cup grapefruit juice (I like to use pink grapefruit juice)
- 2 tablespoons of unflavored powdered gelatin
- 1 tablespoon of mint-infused honey (refer to instructions for creating infused honey later in this chapter)

To begin making CBD gummies: in a small saucepan, over medium-low heat, add fruit juice. Add gelatin and honey. Stir frequently until the gelatin and honey are completely dissolved. Remove from heat.

Mix in CBD oil (or CBD isolate powder.) Stir until fully incorporated.

Place gummy molds on a cookie sheet tray on a flat surface. The cookie sheet will help you easily transfer the molds to the refrigerator. Use a spoon to fill each gummy mold with liquid mixture. Stir mixture occasionally while filling molds.

Place gummy molds in the refrigerator. Be sure molds are lying flat for best results. Refrigerate for thirty minutes or until mixture fully sets.

Remove gummies from molds and store in an airtight container in the refrigerator for up to two weeks.

If you're looking for an even faster, fun way to make a fruit-flavored dissolvable CBD snack, try adding your CBD oil to fruit-flavored gelatin (like Jello). Prepare your gelatin per normal, divide gelatin evenly into compartments of a silicone ice-cube tray. Stir in a single 1/2 ml or 1 ml dose of CBD oil into each portion.

Place ice-cube tray(s) in refrigerator. Chill and set gelatin per package directions. Pop out a gelatin cube to enjoy as needed. Cubes may be stored in covered ice-cube trays (or an airtight container) in refrigerator for up to two weeks.

CBD FOOD-PAIRING IDEAS

The same as when pairing herbs with foods, use your taste buds as the guide. Not all CBD oils are created equal. Some have a smoother, milder taste profile and some will be more pungent and herbaceous.

Remember when we discussed terpenes in Chapter 2? To refresh your memory, terpenes are organic compounds that give plants, flowers, and herbs their unique aromas, colors, and flavors.

Some fans of cannabis enjoy seeking a particular flavor profile for food via terpenes. A current trend is to match the predominant terpene present in the CBD flowers or oil you're cooking with to ingredients containing the same terpene.

For example, if the CBD oil you're using has a detectable note of the terpene Linalool present, a few ingredients for the recipe that would pair well would be thyme, coriander, and lemon juice. Thyme, coriander, and lemon peel (citrus) all naturally contain the terpene Linalool.

If this is a technique you're interested in, you can use the following chart for ideas on ingredients that naturally contain the same prominent terpenes that cannabis plants often contain:

TERPENE	PAIRS WELL WITH
Limonene	basil, celeriac, citrus, dill, fennel, peppermint, rosemary, spearmint
Myrcene	basil, bay, cardamom, hops, lemongrass, mangos, oregano, parsley, rosemary, sage, thyme
Nerolidol	basil, cardamom, ginger, lavender, lemongrass, peppers, tarragon
Alpha-Pinene + Beta-Pinene	dill, lemon balm, nutmeg, orange peel, rosemary, turmeric

TERPENE	PAIRS WELL WITH (cont.)
Linalool	basil, bee balm, citrus, coriander, lavender, marjoram, mint, oregano, rose, thyme
Humulene	basil, clove, ginseng, ginger, hops, pepper, sage
Terpineol	apples, cumin, lilac, mint, nutmeg
Caryophyllene	black pepper, cinnamon, clove, oregano

How do you know what terpenes are prominent in your CBD oil? You should be able to quickly locate this information on the manufacturer's website or in the lab testing report. (Refer to the "Lab Testing" section in Chapter 3 to help you locate and interpret lab testing results.)

The same applies if you're purchasing cannabis flowers with a high concentration of CBD for use in cooking. Sellers should have the terpene profile listed in the description of the flower, and you should be able to locate percentages contained on the lab testing results. If you are purchasing via a dispensary, the staff should be able to help you navigate and find strains with the terpene profile you're most interested in.

When in doubt about what terpenes your full-spectrum CBD oil contains, you may be able to count on Limonene being prominent. According to Science Direct, "Limonene is one of the most abundant terpenes in cannabis, and it may be found in concentrations as high as 16 percent of the essential oil fraction."[40]

Matching terpenes in your CBD oil to other ingredients in your recipes can be a fun and flavorful way to enhance the taste of your recipes and boost the effects of the terpene(s) in the CBD. Do keep in mind, though, that you can play with terpenes in your recipes without using CBD. The herbs and foods with similar terpenes to those found in cannabis are generally far less expensive than CBD.

If you're attracted to the citrus aroma and the anti-anxiety effects associated with the terpene Limonene, you may find that incorporating ingredients like basil, grapefruit (citrus), or rosemary regularly into your recipes is helpful, without the need for adding in a dose of CBD.

MY FIVE FAVORITE RECIPES FOR ADDING CBD

Now that you have a good understanding of how and why you may want to add CBD to your recipes, here are a few tasty recipes to get you started. Each of these are recipes I've made regularly for a fun way to add a little extra CBD to my diet, or as an alternative way to enjoy my normal daily dose.

I'm taking you on my personal journey from appetizer to dessert—hopefully you'll find a course that inspires you! Do note that you don't need to add CBD to any of these recipes. Each recipe I'm sharing will still turn out lovely even without the addition of CBD.

If you'd like to make an entire five-course meal using this recipe mix, you can just pick one of the recipes to add your daily dose of CBD to, and omit it from the other four recipes.

Garden Salad with CBD Honey Tarragon Dressing

Yield: 4 servings

As many of my personal recipes are, this salad is derived from the Irish cuisine of my childhood and adult travels to the Isle. This style salad makes use of ingredients you're likely to find in any Irish kitchen garden or pantry.

If you prefer other produce in your salad in addition to the ones I've listed, such as tomatoes, add them in. Also feel free to omit any of the produce I've suggested from your salad to create your own custom version.

Ingredients:

4 cups leaf lettuce, rough chopped
2 cups arugula, rough chopped
4 radishes, sliced thin
1 cup cucumber, diced
1 cup cooked or pickled beets, diced
1 hard-boiled egg, cut into eight wedges

Dressing ingredients:

1 teaspoon fresh tarragon, minced
1 tablespoon honey
1/4 cup white wine vinegar
1 teaspoon Dijon mustard
1/4 cup extra-virgin olive oil
salt
CBD oil

To make this salad: in a large mixing bowl, add lettuce, arugula, cucumbers, radishes, and beets. Toss gently until ingredients are fully distributed through salad.

Evenly divide salad between four salad bowls. Top each salad bowl with two egg wedges.

In a small mixing bowl, add vinegar, mustard, and a pinch of salt. Whisk until fully combined.

Add honey. Whisk until fully incorporated.

Add oil and tarragon. Whisk until fully incorporated.

Divide salad dressing evenly between four small glass jars or cups. I typically use shot glasses to separate the portions.

Add 1/2 to 1 ml of CBD oil in your preferred dose to each salad dressing cup.

Prior to pouring dressing over each salad portion, use a swizzle stick or the handle of a spoon to gently stir the dressing to incorporate the CBD oil.

GRILLED PEACHES WITH CBD AND HONEY RICOTTA

Yield: 4 servings

Great as an appetizer, dessert, or snack, this recipe combines sweet and savory beautifully. It's ideal in the summertime, but equally enjoyable in winter. If you don't feel like grilling, you can simply warm some canned peach halves in a skillet and then top with the ricotta mix prior to serving.

Ingredients:

2 fresh peaches, halved with pit removed

1/2 cup ricotta cheese

1 tablespoon honey

8 fresh basil leaves, chopped

CBD

Decide how many milligrams of CBD you would like to have in each serving of grilled peaches. Multiple that number by four (the number of servings) to determine how many milligrams total of CBD to add to your recipe. (For additional help, refer to the instructions and chart featured in the "Best Methods for Using CBD in Recipes" section earlier in this chapter.)

Preheat grill to medium heat. Place peach on the grill, inside (cut side) down. Grill two to three minutes or until grill marks appear and fruit is beginning to soften.

Use tongs or a spatula to flip peach over, bottom side (skin side) on grill. Grill for three to four minutes or until the fruit is completely softened. Remove from grill and set peach halves aside.

In a small bowl, add ricotta cheese, honey, and CBD oil. Stir until ingredients are distributed well and thoroughly combined.

Divide ricotta into four equal portions. Top each peach half with a portion of the ricotta mix. Garnish each portion with chopped basil and serve.

CBD-INFUSED GARLIC MASHED POTATOES

Yield: 10 servings

Potatoes are one of my ultimate comfort foods. I use this quick, easy recipe regularly. The boost of garlic is an awesome way to infuse more medicinal garden goodness into your day, and it overpowers any trace of CBD oil taste in the recipe.

To me, garlic and CBD have a harmonious relationship, too, as they are both anti-inflammatories that provide additional health and wellness benefits.

Ingredients:
3 pounds of potatoes (I prefer to
    use Yukon Gold potatoes),
    peeled and cut into quarters
2 cups heavy cream
4 cloves garlic, minced
1 teaspoon garlic powder
CBD oil
salt and black pepper

To begin, first determine how many milligrams of CBD you ideally want to have in each portion of mashed potatoes. Multiple that number by ten (the number of servings) to determine how many milligrams total of CBD to add to your recipe. (For additional help, refer to the instructions and chart featured in the "Best Methods for Using CBD in Recipes" section earlier in this chapter.) Take into consideration whether you're likely to eat more than one serving of this tasty dish at a time!

Place the peeled and quartered potatoes into a large saucepan. Fill saucepan with water until it fully covers the potatoes.

Cook over a high heat until water comes to a boil. Reduce heat to medium to maintain rolling boil. Cook for twenty-five to thirty minutes or until potatoes are soft (they will fall apart when gently pressed with a fork).

Remove from heat. Drain off the water from the potatoes. Reserve 1/4 cup of water.

Gently mash potatoes. Add cream, garlic, garlic powder, and CBD oil. Continue to mash potatoes until all ingredients are fully incorporated. If potatoes are too thick, add a tablespoon of reserved water at a time while you continue mashing to thin potatoes to desired consistency.

Add salt and pepper to potatoes, to taste. Stir mashed potatoes thoroughly to ensure an even distribution of all ingredients. Portion and serve.

GRILLED CHICKEN WITH FRESH CBD MARINARA

Yield: 1 serving

This humble dish is a fast, easy, and flavorful lunch or light dinner meal. Pair it with the CBD-infused garlic mashed potatoes for a complete meal. (Again, you can omit the CBD from any recipe to ensure you do not dose more than you want in your meal.)

There are plenty of ways to prep chicken, but there's something to be said for the sheer simplicity of this dish, which beautifully showcases the purity of farm fresh flavors.

Ingredients:

1 4-ounce boneless chicken
*   breast without skin*
1/4 cup tomato, diced
1 small clove garlic, minced
2 fresh basil leaves, minced
1/4 teaspoon dried oregano
1 tablespoon extra-virgin olive oil
your preferred dose of CBD oil
*   (1/2 ml to 1 ml serving)*

In a small mixing bowl, add tomato, garlic, basil, oregano, olive oil, and CBD oil. Stir gently until ingredients are evenly distributed. Set aside.

Rub both sides of chicken breast with a pinch of salt and black pepper.

Using your preferred method (using your outdoor grill or a small skillet on your stovetop), grill chicken for approximately four to five minutes per side until done. When a safe minimum temperature is reached, remove chicken from grill. (You can find more information about safe minimum cooking temperatures for meat on the U.S. Department of Agriculture website at usda.gov.) Always err on the side of safety, as undercooked chicken is not safe to eat. If you do not own a meat thermometer, it's an excellent investment to purchase one.

Plate chicken. Gently stir marina mix to refresh and ensure ingredients are evenly distributed. Pour marina mix over chicken and serve.

CARDAMOM ROSE CBD MUG CAKE

Yield: two 8-ounce mug cakes

Loosely based on a cake I enjoyed at a Persian coffee house once, this recipe is a great way to begin your CBD edibles experience, as it's a small batch recipe. This allows you to experiment a little without committing to baking a full cake.

You'll notice it makes great use of some medicinal garden goodies like wild roses and cardamom, too. Cardamom, rose, and CBD all have lovely stress-relieving properties, making this a great dessert to help end your day on a mellow note.

Ingredients:

2 tablespoons butter, softened
2 tablespoons almond milk
6 tablespoons self-rising flour
2 teaspoons rose water (recipe in Chapter 8)
1 egg
1/4 cup sugar
1/4 teaspoon powdered cardamom
1/2 to 1 ml of CBD oil with your preferred dose (do not add more than 1 ml of CBD oil)
salt

To create cardamom rose CBD mug cakes, in a small mixing bowl, cream butter and sugar with a beater (or fork) until smooth.

Add rose water, egg, CBD oil, and almond milk. Stir until ingredients are fully incorporated.

Add flour, cardamom, and a small pinch of salt. Beat with a beater (or fork) until batter is smooth.

Divide batter evenly between two eight-to-ten-ounce mugs.

Insert one mug into the microwave. Microwave for two minutes or until cake rises and is firm without visible wet spots. If there are still wet spots visible, microwave for ten second intervals (checking cake every ten seconds) until cake is fully firm and no wet spots in the batter remain. Remove cake from microwave and set aside.

Repeat microwave process with second cake. Remove cake from microwave. Allow cakes to cool for two minutes. Serve and enjoy!

If you want to dress things up, add a dollop of whipped cream on top and sprinkle on a few chopped black walnuts or pistachio nuts.

FRESH-BAKED TIP: A super easy way to add CBD to your premade desserts like brownies, cakes, or ice cream is to whip up a quick thin ganache to drizzle on top using CBD-infused chocolates (or regular chocolate with a bit of CBD oil).

To create a ganache drizzle, you will need:

- 2 ounces of CBD-infused milk or dark chocolate in your preferred dose (you should be easily able to identify the dose per ounce of CBD chocolate bar on the product label)
- 2 tablespoons heavy cream

OR

- 2 ounces of milk or dark chocolate (chunk of bar or chocolate chips)
- 2 tablespoons heavy cream
- 1/2 to 1 ml of CBD oil in preferred dose (do not use more than 1 ml for this recipe)

In a small microwave-safe bowl, add cream and CBD chocolate (or regular chocolate).

Microwave on high for fifteen seconds. Remove and stir. Continue microwaving at ten-second intervals, removing bowl and stirring ingredients until chocolate is fully melted and cream is fully incorporated. If the mixture is too thick, add a little extra cream to thin.

If you used regular chocolate, once the chocolate is fully melted and mixed with the cream, add the CBD oil and stir it into the chocolate ganache until it's fully incorporated.

Drizzle ganache over a brownie, slice of cake, ice cream, sliced strawberries, or other preferred single portion desserts.

HOW TO MAKE HERB BUTTER

From seasoning popcorn to finishing steaks off the grill, fresh herb butter is an awesome tool to have in your culinary kit. It's a great way to make use of fresh medicinal garden herbs and to add more of them to your diet.

Herb butter can be substituted in any recipe or cooking method that calls for butter. You can also use it as a spread for bread and bakery goods.

Note: You can use butter alternatives for creating herb butter, if preferred, like light butters or plant-based butter spreads.

To make herb butter, it's best to soften the butter to room temperature first. Use two tablespoons of fresh, clean, chopped herbs per four-ounce stick of butter. Rosemary is the go-to herb for butters, as it pairs well with so many dishes and is ridiculously delicious as a bread spread. I whip up a basil and oregano butter regularly for use with Italian-inspired dishes and to use for garlic breads.

In a mixing bowl, use a hand mixer (or a fork and some elbow power) to cream butter. Add herbs. Gently fold in herbs until evenly distributed.

Use a spatula to shape butter into a circle or oblong shape. Store in refrigerator in an airtight container. Portion off a chunk as needed.

Alternatively, you can mold herb butter into pre-set portions using a silicone ice-cube tray. For fun, you can also shape butter portions using candy molds or silicone shape molds (found at craft stores and online). Rosemary butter pads shaped like pumpkins are a super cute and delicious addition to your Thanksgiving holiday table!

After mixing the butter and herbs, press the herb butter portions into the ice-cube tray or shape molds. Refrigerate for two hours.

Pop butter shapes from the molds, store in the refrigerator in an airtight container, and use as needed.

CREATING MEDICINAL GARDEN HONEY MIXES

Medicinal garden honey mixtures can be used as daily supplements or as an elixir. A teaspoon of thyme-infused honey is great for soothing an irritated throat and quieting coughs.

Flavored honeys are also wonderful for using as a sugar substitute in recipes, adding to salad dressings, or drizzling over desserts.

If you have allergies, do be mindful of using honey elixirs, as they can trigger an allergic reaction. Bees collect pollen from many plant sources. If honey isn't already a part of your normal diet, proceed with caution.

There are two methods I use to infuse honey with medicinal garden plants:

1. I mix powered spices directly with honey to immediately infuse.
2. I steep dried herbs in honey to infuse flavor and plant properties over time.

For powdered spices, simply measure out the amount of powdered spice (like ginger or turmeric) that you want to use for a dose or recipe and add honey to it until it forms a paste. In the medicinal plant world, this process is called creating an "electuary."

Consume honey paste "as is," add it to a recipe, or add to eight ounces of hot water to enjoy a soothing cup of medicinal tea.

You can make larger portions of electuary and store them for regular use, for up to one month. Store in a labeled airtight container in a cool, dry, dark spot.

Measure out your desired amount (for example, one teaspoon) as needed.

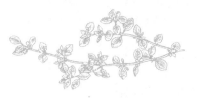

HERB-INFUSED HONEY

Mint-infused or lemon-balm infused honeys are my preferred sweetener of choice to use with most medicinal teas throughout the year.

To create, you'll need two glass jars with a tight seal.

Tip: Clean and save your old honey jars to repurpose for this recipe.

Fill a honey jar halfway with your dried herb of choice. Do not use fresh herbs, only use dried. Fresh herbs will have a trace of water present and this can lead to bacteria growth.

Pour honey over dried herbs until the jar is filled. Tap jar gently and/or swirl contents to ensure herbs are coated with honey.

Note: If the jar has a small opening, use a funnel to help you fill the jar with herbs and honey.

Seal jar and label. Place jar in a cool, dark, dry spot for two weeks. Each day turn the jar over to ensure herbs are well coated with honey while infusing.

After the two-week period, use a fine mesh strainer (and funnel, if needed) to strain honey into a clean jar. Label jar and store in a cool, dark, dry space. Use as needed.

When stored properly, honey typically remains fresh for up to two years. Infused honey has the same shelf life. If your infused honey starts to get cloudy and/or begins to crystalize, it's best to properly dispose of it.

Herbs leftover after straining can be used within a few days in salad dressings and marinades, or to create herbal teas.

For herbal tea, simply portion some of the honey-coated herbs into a mesh tea strainer and steep in boiling hot water for five to fifteen minutes (depending upon desired strength of tea).

There are CBD-infused honey products on the market now, too, for use with herbal tea. You'll find out more about them in Chapter 8.

FRESH-BAKED TIP: Herbs leftover from making rosemary-infused honey can be used to create the Honey Lemon Rosemary Facial Mask for normal-to-oily skin featured in my prior book, *Getting Laid: Everything You Need to Know About Raising Chickens, Gardening and Preserving.*

In a small bowl, add one tablespoon of lemon juice and three tablespoons of the strained rosemary honey coated herbs. Stir until ingredients are fully mixed. Warm mix in the microwave for ten seconds or until warm to the touch.

Spread a thin layer across your face, avoiding eye area, mouth, and nose openings. Leave on for thirty minutes, then wash off with warm water to enjoy your glowing skin!

Another great way to use herb-infused honey and dried spices from your medicinal garden is to make your own mustard for use in salad dressings and recipes, or as a traditional sandwich spread.

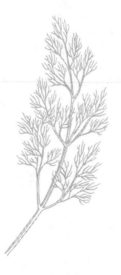

DILL HONEY MUSTARD

Yield: 6 ounces

Ingredients:
1/2 cup mustard powder
6 tablespoons cider vinegar
1 teaspoon turmeric powder
1/4 teaspoon paprika powder
1/8 teaspoon garlic paste
1 tablespoon dill-infused honey
1/2 teaspoon salt
purified water

In a small saucepan over a medium-high heat (or via use of a tea kettle), bring 1/4 cup of water to a boil. Remove from heat.

In a small mixing bowl, add mustard powder. Pour in boiling water and stir until mixture forms a paste.

Add vinegar, whisk until smooth. Add turmeric, salt, paprika, and garlic paste. Whisk until smooth.

Stir in dill-infused honey until fully incorporated into mustard mix.

Cover the bowl with a lid or saran wrap. Store in a dark, dry space for twenty-four hours.

After twenty-four hours, open container and thoroughly stir ingredients. Pour mustard into a glass jar. Seal tightly and store in refrigerator for up to one month.

Tip: If you like hot mustard with more kick, store the bowl at room temperature for three to five days, checking daily to test the heat level until your desired flavor is achieved. Once the mustard is spicy enough for your taste, thoroughly stir ingredients and pour mustard into a glass jar. Seal jar tightly, and store in refrigerator for up to one month.

HEMPSEEDS, HEMP FLOUR, AND HEMP PROTEIN POWDERS

In Chapter 2, we briefly touched on all the merits of the cannabis plant that extend past compounds like CBD and THC.

Food-grade hempseeds (also called "hemp hearts" when shelled) contain only minute traces of CBD, so they are not a solution for medicinal dosing, but they are a wonderful nutritional powerhouse ingredient worth considering. Adding them to your diet may aid your overall health and wellness needs.

Hempseeds are:

- full of plant-based protein
- gluten-free
- chock full of fiber
- rich with essential fatty acids like omega 3, omega 6, and gamma linolenic acid (GLA)
- vegan-friendly
- KETO-friendly
- high in magnesium, vitamin E, potassium, calcium, zinc, and iron

With a mild nut-like flavor, hempseeds can be sprinkled on yogurt, oatmeal, salads, and even desserts. They are well loved in smoothies, smoothie bowls, and home-made granola bars. You can also munch on them by the handful.

Hemp protein powder and hemp flour, which are derived from hempseeds, have the same attributes, including the mild nutty flavor. Because of the way they are processed, however, hemp protein powders and hemp flour generally have less essential fatty acids than hempseeds.

When using hemp flour in recipes, it will give the recipe a nutty, earthy flavor. This translates well into most baked goods, especially breads.

Hemp protein powder is most often used for creating smoothies, smoothie bowls, or shakes and as an additive to oatmeal and cereals. Many hempseed, hemp flour, and hemp protein powder products are currently sourced from or manufactured outside of the United States.

Prior to purchasing, check out the company's website and find out where the plant is sourced. Like every health and wellness ingredient, investigate to ensure you are purchasing a quality, pure product from a source you trust. With their "Sourced Non-GMO Pledge," I've found Bob's Red Mill hempseed products to be of good quality. Nutiva offers U.S.-grown organic hempseed products, and I've also found them to be a good source of quality products.

As my husband has high cholesterol, hempseeds with their high levels of good fatty acids are a good dietary choice for him. He typically sprinkles them on oatmeal in the morning for a daily dose.

Another way I found to help him include hempseeds is to incorporate them into his snack time with homemade hempseed and oat granola bars. Granola bars in the grocery store are often high in sugar and saturated fats. When you DIY, you can control your ingredients and create a better-for-you, all-natural version.

Making your own granola bars is easy, and if you've never tried a fresh, home-made granola bar, you are truly in for a treat!

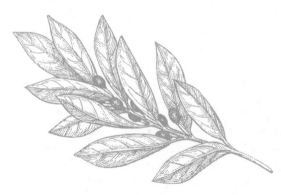

HEMPSEED AND OAT GRANOLA BARS

Yield: 10–12 servings

Ingredients:

2 cups organic rolled oats
1 cup organic quick-cooking oats
1/2 teaspoon cinnamon
1/8 teaspoon salt
1/4 cup raw almond slices
  (can substitute other nuts, if
  preferred)
1 tablespoon extra-virgin olive oil
  (or sunflower oil)
1/3 cup pure maple syrup
1/4 cup honey
1/4 cup almond milk
1/4 cup of hempseeds or hemp
  hearts
Optional: 1/4 cup raisins
Optional: 1/4 cup shredded
  coconut

Preheat oven to 350 degrees Fahrenheit.

Process two cups of rolled oats in blender or food processor until they become flour-like. Mix "oat flour" with all dry ingredients (except coconut) in a bowl.

Add all wet ingredients to the dry mixture and stir until well combined.

Optional: gently fold raisins into mixture.

In a nine-inch by twelve-inch glass (or nonstick) baking dish, add mixture to the dish. Press mixture down until you have a flat layer that is about half-inch in height.

Optional: Sprinkle coconut on top.

Using a butter knife, cut flattened mixture into ten to twelve equal size bars.

Bake granola bars for fifteen minutes, or until lightly browned. Remove from oven.

Cool on cooling rack for fifteen minutes. Using your original cut lines, recut the bar shapes and break bars apart.

If you leave them on the counter and you have a big family or hungry teenagers like I do, they will disappear within the day! Otherwise, store in an airtight container in a cool, dry, dark space for up to two weeks. Use as needed.

CBD-INFUSED FOODS AND TRAVEL

With CBD popping up in edible forms, CBD oil considered a liquid supplement, and various laws regarding cannabis products throughout the United States and internationally, it's important to be in tune with travel restrictions.

For air travel, the best resource is the Transportation Security Administration (TSA). You can find up-to-date lists of what is and is not allowed to bring on an airplane at tsa.gov.

It's equally important to research the laws regarding cannabis products and prescriptions for each state or country you're traveling to. It may be acceptable and legal to bring the products on an airplane, but once you leave the plane, you need to know what to expect.

Currently, around twenty states in the United States have no hemp-derived cannabidiol product restrictions, but that means around thirty states do. Some states only allow CBD use with a prescription.

Some countries don't allow cannabis-derived products in any form. The federal government also has laws regarding transportation of cannabidiol products.

Weedmaps.com is a good resource to start with to determine the cannabis laws inside and outside of the United States.

Because of the varied restrictions, a new travel trend call "cannatourism" is gaining popularity. Travelers from various countries or states where cannabis products are not legal for recreational use are traveling to areas where it is legal. Wherever you're traveling, for whatever reason, whether it be by car, cruise ship, or train, you should still research and clearly understand the laws for every location you'll be visiting.

If you have a prescription for a cannabis product, bring a copy of it with you. If you're using an OTC product, print off a copy of the lab report for the product and bring it with you. This way, in case your CBD oil is questioned by a TSA agent or local authority, you can help address the concerns with supportive, credible documentation.

Rethink traveling with edibles, like chocolates you purchase or cookies you bake. They could cause flags to be raised during security screening at the airport, and you won't have any proof to provide justification for their legal transport. Another way to avoid complications with airport security or law enforcement in states you are driving through is to purchase CBD products when you arrive at your destination (provided they are legally sold within the state or country you're visiting).

A FEW MORE NOTES ON CBD-INFUSED FOODS

Cannabis cooking has had a big boom. If you're curious about cannabinoids and food, you don't need to look further than your television, internet, or local bookstore.

We are at the beginning of an extremely exciting time. The global hemp industry is poised to change many product categories, including dietary supplements and food. You're going to see more and more cannabis recipes and products as the market evolves and regulations change.

Does CBD have to be in every product you consume?

Nope.

Too much, as the saying goes, can be too much. You wouldn't want to fill your coffee mug with more liquid than it can hold, would you?

If consuming 10 mg of full-spectrum CBD every day to help ease your anxiety works for you, then there's no need to add more to your daily consumption. It's just overflowing your individual cup.

Adding foods and drinks infused with CBD to your daily diet could easily up your dosage by five to ten times more than you normally consume. This won't increase the effectiveness of your dose if your dose is already working—but, it may increase the amount you spend on CBD per day, and it could give you some less desirable outcomes like making you sleepy or increasing your appetite.

There's nothing wrong with the notion of finding alternative ways for adding CBD to your diet, especially if you're finding the properties to be of high benefit to your overall health and wellness. It's simply important to ask how much CBD you truly need to consume, and to demand answers on the science of CBD edibles from chefs and companies producing edibles.

In our own homes, some of the beneficial aspects of creating your own CBD-infused product options, like coffees or cookies, is that doing so offers you more choices in delivery method and gives you full dosage control. Enjoying a piece of homemade gourmet CBD-infused chocolate at the end of a full day can be a pleasurable way to get your daily dose (provided this delivery method works for you).

This can be a key element of easily incorporating CBD into your lifestyle. The flexibility of having alternative dosing options can make it easier to make your holistic approach a habit, not a chore.

Be wary of CBD cookbooks. If you are interested in new recipes, they may have some good ideas, but there's no real trick to adding CBD to your smoothie or daily meal, and there's no science to back up whether it's an effective delivery method (as you've already discovered in this chapter).

There are some amazing chefs who are experimenting with infusing cannabis into your dining experience. Most are in tune with the science of cooking, understanding ways in which cannabis may elevate a dish or compliment a flavor profile. When you pick up a CBD cookbook, ask yourself if the author has done the research, if they can back up any claims with credible resources, and if the recipes will enhance your lifestyle in a reasonable and affordable way.

There's just not a need to overdo it. Once you've achieved your optimum CBD dose, adding more isn't necessarily better.

It's also important to use your savvy shopping skills as a consumer and be aware of industry standards. If a food is USDA Organic approved, it will typically have the USDA Organic certification seal displayed on the package.[41] We are used to seeing other certifications on products, such as "Fair Trade Certified," awarded to companies who meet "rigorous social, environmental, and economic standards."[42] Look for these types of assurances, too, when you are considering the purchase of CBD products in the future.

A promising new certification for food, fiber, and personal care ingredients, anticipated to launch in 2021, is the Regenerative Organic Certified (ROC) program. This is the exciting one to watch for with hemp products, as it means the farms producing the plant and the manufacturer producing products both "meet the highest standards for soil health, animal welfare, and farmworker fairness."[43] (Learn more about this initiative at regenorganic.org.)

Purchasing products that are not regulated is a gamble, at best. Odds are it will be likely to be a waste of your resources, including your financial ones.

Brewing Medicinal Teas, Custom Coffees, Smoothies, Cocktails, and CBD infusions

One of the quickest, easiest, and most refreshing ways to enjoy your medicinal garden is to use your herbs and spices to create or infuse beverages.

You can easily add your CBD oil into these beverages, too, for a one-cup elixir of aromatic, flavor-filled health and wellness joy!

MAKING MEDICINAL GARDEN TEAS

Every herb, spice, and edible flower in this guide, with the exceptions of comfrey and aloe, can be used to create a medicinal tea, or as it is referred to in the herbalist world, a "tisane."

Comfrey is toxic to humans when consumed orally. *Do not* use it in your medicinal teas.

Aloe gel from the interior of the leaves can be used to create aloe water, but it has a very distinct flavor and texture that many people do not enjoy. Plus, aloe vera, when consumed, is known to cause allergic reactions.

Also take note that any medicinal plant can trigger allergies or interfere with medicines you are already taking. Always consult your preferred medical professionals before starting a medicinal tea regimen.

Why do people love herbal teas? Along with exceptional flavor, they also have mild natural remedy properties. Mint is a well-known digestive aid, chamomile is often used as a sleep aid, and lavender may help calm your nerves.

Herbal teas are not true teas, as they do not contain traditional tea leaves harvested from the tea plant (*Camellia sinensis*).

Medicinal teas differ from herbal teas in two significant ways:

1. **Medicinal teas are strong brews.** Steeping time is thirty minutes or more.

2. **The intent of medicinal tea is therapeutic.** You may (and *should*) enjoy the aromatics and flavor of a medicinal tea, but it's brewed specifically to support a health concern you have.

Before you create a medicinal tea, you will need to gather several items:

- **fresh and/or dried herbs and spices**—you'll need one tablespoon of fresh herbs/spices/flowers per one cup of water. If you're using dried herbs/spices/flowers, you'll need one teaspoon of dried herbs/spices/flowers per one cup of water
- **purified water**—water that has not been purified may taint the tea with trace elements and minerals, which will affect the outcome and may result in a more bitter tea
- **large tea pot with strainer**—or a large saucepan and fine mesh strainer

To make medicinal tea, bring water to a boil. Add medicinal plants to water. Steep for thirty to sixty minutes.

The longer you steep, the stronger the taste will be, so you may want to experiment and adjust your timing accordingly. At a minimum, steep for thirty minutes to infuse as much of the plant's properties into the water as possible.

Strain medicinal plants from the tisane you just created. Pour a cup of the medicinal tea, rewarm it in the tea pot or microwave. Sip and enjoy.

The remainder of the tea may be stored in a glass jar in the refrigerator and used over the next one to two days. To use, reheat the tea or enjoy it in an iced tea form.

Note: Seeds and root spices may need a longer steep. Add them to your tea pot when you fill the pot with water, prior to applying heat for boil.

If you just want to enjoy one cup of tea and don't want a larger batch, you can use a cup-size tea strainer. Simply fill the strainer with your preferred fresh and/ or dried ingredients, place in a teacup, and pour boiling water directly into the teacup. Steep for thirty minutes (or longer). Then, remove strainer and reheat tea in microwave to warm.

If you plan to use dry ingredients for your medicinal tea regularly, you can premake tea bag packets for ease of use. Ideally, you'll want to use all-natural, unbleached, chlorine-free tea bags. You can find these for sale at your local organic grocer or online, typically in a-hundred-count (or higher) packages for a modest cost.

Portion out your dried ingredients into each bag, seal, and store bags in an airtight container in a cool, dry, dark space. Use as needed.

You can add honey, herbal-infused honey (recipe in Chapter 7), maple syrup, cream, or other sweeteners to your medicinal tea, if preferred, to mellow the taste and make it a more enjoyable experience for you each day.

Use the charts provided in Chapters 4 and 5 to select herbs and spices for your medicinal teas to aid with specific ailments. Combine them for flavor enhancement. For example, fennel with ginger and turmeric is a lovely blend to use for aid with digestive issues like heartburn, bloating, nausea, and gas. For a pick-me-up to help you focus, try a combination of peppermint, spearmint, and rosemary. Add a touch of honey to help balance these strong flavors. Stressed out? Brew a blend of catnip, cinnamon, and lemon balm.

Medicinal teas certainly don't have to be boring! Experiment with flavors until you find the ones that work and taste the best.

DOS AND DON'TS FOR USING FRESH INGREDIENTS FOR MEDICINAL TEAS

DO pick fresh ingredients directly prior to brewing. For spices like ginger, grate fresh just before you brew.

DON'T use any plants that have been sprayed with fertilizer, pesticides, or any other chemicals.

DO remove dirt and any other debris from fresh ingredients prior to brewing.

DO crush leaves or petals for fresh plants gently with your fingertips to help release oils prior to making your medicinal tea.

DON'T assume fresh (or dried) herbs you purchase for supplemental use are free of toxins like pesticide sprays. Investigate prior to purchasing. Interview the farmer at the farmer's market to find out their planting and harvesting practices. Read through the producer's website to learn how the plants are sourced and cultivated.

HOW MUCH MEDICINAL TEA SHOULD I DRINK?

With medicinal teas and tinctures, how do you know what dose to take? Just as we discussed with CBD use, start with a low dose, and slowly introduce the herb or spice into your medicinal routine.

When you make a medicinal tea or tincture, start with a few sips, and see how you feel. Note your reactions. If you are doing well, slowly increase your amount. Every person has different supplemental needs. There's no precise prescription when it comes to determining how much medicinal tea you need each day.

You may decide one cup of medicinal tea in the morning each day is the perfect amount to address your health concerns. Perhaps you may need multiple medicinal teas and tinctures throughout the day to address various aspects of your wellness routine, from increasing focus to enhancing sleep. Some medicinal teas or tinctures you will only need once a year, such as peppermint tea to help with indigestion after a large holiday meal.

A typical dose for medicinal tea is eight ounces, and a typical dose of an herbal tincture is one teaspoon, but that may be too much or too little for you. It will take some effort on your part to begin with a small dose and increase over time until you achieve the effect you desire, but it will be well worth the effort when the effects are positive ones!

The key is time. Like CBD, medicinal herbs and spices may take a few weeks to reveal their results. They aren't a one-dose magical cure-all, especially if you're dealing with chronic issues. For sudden issues like a stomachache, they can help you quickly resolve matters, but if you have a consistent chronic health concern, steady regular use of a tincture over time will better help support your health needs.

Cooking with herbs and spices can be done regularly and in pretty much any dose you desire. Most herbs and spices are tolerated very well in high doses. Your body will use what it needs and flush out the rest.

Some, however, when used in concentrated forms will cause immediate reactions. Remember the cinnamon challenge craze on social media a few years ago? People found out quickly, a mouthful of cinnamon produced awful side effects. Cinnamon is an extraordinarily strong spice—a little goes a long way in providing excellent flavor and health benefits.

Many years ago, I started adding fennel seeds to my medicinal tea brew. Fennel seeds are often useful as an anti-inflammatory and digestive aid—both properties that suit my health and wellness needs well. About a month later, I started breaking out in hives. After ruling out many other factors, I discovered it was the fennel seed causing my reaction. Hives and rashes are a known potential side effect of fennel seed use.

The initial effect of adding the fennel seeds to my medicinal tea was great, but over time, my body developed an intolerance. Always listen to your body, and don't dismiss discomforts, signs of allergic reactions, or anything that you deem problematic. Like me, you may not have a reaction to an herb or spice at first but can later develop intolerances.

WebMD (webmd.com) is a decent resource for checking out potential herb and spice side effects prior to using them. You'll find a comprehensive listing under the "Drugs & Supplements" section of the website.

I've included a Medicinal Garden Tracker chart on the next page to help you track your reactions. (You can also find a printable download version of the chart at ruralmom.com/getting-baked). Use it daily to make notes of your dosage amounts and the results. After a few weeks, review your results and adjust your routine, as needed.

Medicinal Garden Tracker

Herb/Spice:
Delivery Form:
Date:
Dose:
Results:

Herb/Spice:
Delivery Form:
Date:
Dose:
Results:

Herb/Spice:
Delivery Form:
Date:
Dose:
Results:

Herb/Spice:
Delivery Form:
Date:
Dose:
Results:

FRESH-BAKED TIP: You can use your medicinal tea bags for herbal baths, too!

Tea bags help you contain plant particles for less clean up later. Fill tea bag with fresh and/or dried ingredients. Secure the top of the tea bag with string, tying tightly to prevent any leaking of the ingredients.

Hold the filled tea bag under warm running water just as you begin to fill your bathtub, until it is soaked through. Next, place the bag in the bath water to steep as your bathtub is filling.

Once the bathtub is full, you can remove the bag prior to taking your bath or leave it in for continued aromatics. Just remember to remove the tea bag at the end of your bath prior to draining the tub.

CBD IN YOUR MEDICINAL TEA

If you're seeking an alternative way to use your morning or evening dose of CBD oil, you can simply add it to your medicinal tea.

After the tea is brewed and rewarmed, ready for your enjoyment, add your CBD oil to the tea and give it a stir. Drink and savor the experience.

Another alternative is to add a CBD honey stick to your medicinal tea. For this product, CBD is extracted from industrial hemp, mixed with honey, and then generally packaged in a sealed straw-like package format identical to traditional liquid honey sticks.

Just like adding CBD oil to foods, adding it to your tea may affect how well your dose is absorbed by your body.

Tea and cannabis expert, and founder of Empress Teas, Bethany Stiles suggests there may be an additional problem with adding CBD oils to medicinal teas. Oil-based CBD tinctures tend to sit on the top of the tea or adhere to the side of the cup.

Resolving this issue, along with her love of medicinal tea and a desire to create a sustainable, organic, CBD-infused tea sourced in the United States, is a huge part of the inspiration that led to the development of Empress Teas (empressteas.com). These flavorful teas currently use a water-soluble CBD isolate for easy absorption by the body and better incorporation into the tea.

Those wanting a full- or broad-spectrum CBD tea may see additional offerings developed by Empress Teas. There are currently other tea companies offering full- and broad-spectrum tea options. As always, use the information in Chapters 2 and 3 to help you determine the quality of the product offered.

The drawback to retail teas, of course, is the preferred medicinal plant blend you want may not be available with a CBD additive. An easy solution is to add one of your own medicinal herbs during the brewing process.

Tea potency of a retail tea may be weaker than a traditional medicinal tea as well, even with additional brew time, as these teas are primarily designed for enjoyment and delivery of CBD.

Absolutely nothing wrong, though, with enjoying a cup or two in addition to your daily medicinal tea!

MAKING MEDICINAL GARDEN WATERS

Typically referred to as herbal waters, medicinal garden water beverages are quick and easy to create.

These are not infused waters, like you often see in spa settings. Spa waters are typically waters where ingredients like fresh mint and cucumber are added to cold water for flavor enhancement. You can certainly add fresh herbs to your glass of water anytime for flavor enhancement, but for medicinal waters, you'll want to extract the plant's full potential.

Like medicinal teas, medicinal waters are intense in flavor and created to address specific health needs. Popular medicinal waters include rose, mint, and lemongrass. They can be enjoyed straight, mixed with soda water, or used as a base for smoothies.

To make medicinal water you will need:

- fresh herbs or flower petals[†]
- purified water
- blender

[†] Make sure that you're never using herbs or flower petals that have been treated with pesticides, fertilizers, or other chemicals.

- large tea kettle or large saucepan (I prefer to use an electric tea kettle for this process)
- pitcher with lid (a two-quart pitcher works best)
- fine mess strainer (or cheesecloth)

Note: Powdered herbs or spices generally do not work well for creating medicinal waters. After cooling, the fine particles will settle to the bottom of the pitcher. If you want to add powdered herbs or spices to your water, simply mix the powdered spice or herb directly prior to consuming.

Dried herbs can be used for creating medicinal waters, but they will not be as effective or have the same quality flavor and beneficial amount of plant oils as fresh herbs deliver.

Add herbs or flower petals to blender.

- For rose water—add one cup of petals per one cup of water you will use.
- For all other fresh herbs and flowers—add one-half cup of herbs per one cup of water.

To create a medicinal garden water, heat water to boil. (For quick reference, a two-quart pitcher holds eight cups of water.)

Pour water into blender. Blend for one minute. Allow herb-water mixture to completely cool for one hour.

Using a fine mesh strainer (or cheesecloth), strain water into a pitcher. Discard plant material (may be used in compost).

Place lid on pitcher and store in refrigerator to use as desired for up to one week.

Optionally, for rose water—pour strained rose water into airtight containers, seal, and store in the back of the refrigerator for use when needed, up to one month.

Medicinal garden waters can also be frozen in ice-cube trays for later use to infuse flavor into drinks. Pour water into a silicone ice-cube tray. Place in freezer and allow cubes to fully freeze.

Remove cubes from ice-cube tray and store in an airtight container in the freezer for up to three months. Remove cubes as needed for use in beverages.

 FRESH-BAKED TIP: Rose water soothes, hydrates, and tones your skin. Pop some in a spray bottle to spritz your face after a shower, in the morning before applying moisturizer, or throughout the day to cool off.

Rose water ice cubes are great for cooling off in the hot summer sun, too. Rub along your skin on face, arms, and legs for a quick cool down that will also help quench your dry skin.

PUCKER UP WITH FLAVORED VINEGAR WATERS

I first discovered the joy of adding flavor-infused vinegars to water on an olive oil tasting tour in Kansas City. Our host poured us a glass of water and suggested we add in a few drops of flavored vinegar. I expected my glass to taste more like pickle juice than a refreshing treat, but I'm always game to try new tastes.

To my delight, the herb and fruit-infused vinegars added a refreshing tang to the water, rather than a sour note.

Of course, if you add more than a few drops, you certainly up the pucker factor. The best way to find the perfect amount for your tastes is to experiment a little.

When I returned home, I began to occasionally use my medicinal herb-infused vinegars in this way. It's a great low-calorie way to add flavor enhancement not only to water, but to juice, soda water, and other carbonated beverages, too.

Refer to Chapter 6 for instructions on how to create medicinal herb-infused vinegars.

MEDICINAL GARDEN SMOOTHIES AND SHAKES

While not necessarily a traditional way to create a medicinal brew, health-conscious folks have been adding herbs and powdered spices to milks for centuries. Smoothies and shakes are just the modern version of this practice.

You can add fresh, dried, or powered herbs and spices, hempseeds, CBD oil, herb-infused honey, medicinal waters, leftover medicinal tea, and even edible flowers from your medicinal garden to your daily smoothie with ease.

Adding CBD oil generally works well with smoothies, but again, it could change the amount of effect the tincture has on your body.

Create a pure medicinal garden smoothie or add in ingredients like yogurt, fruits, and vegetables for flavoring and additional health benefits.

For a nearly pure (apart from the added yogurt) medicinal garden shake, try my favorite combination, which I affectionately call my "sunshine mint smoothie":

BARB'S SUNSHINE MINT SMOOTHIE

Ingredients:

1 cup of mint-infused medicinal water

1/2 cup pure unsweetened vanilla Greek yogurt

1/4 teaspoon ginger powder

1/4 teaspoon turmeric powder

1 tablespoon hempseed

1/2 teaspoon lemon-verbena infused honey (see directions for infusing honey in Chapter 7)

Add all ingredients to blender with a half cup of crushed ice. Blend until smooth.

If smoothie is a little too thick, add additional mint-infused water a few teaspoons at a time and continue to blend until smooth. Pour into a glass and enjoy this quick morning pick-me-up!

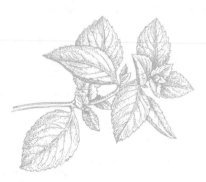

HEMPSEED AND CBD COFFEES—THERAPEUTIC OR JUST TRENDY?

Cannabidiol-infused coffee is popping up at cafes everywhere. The popular sentiment is that CBD coffee will give you the benefit of alertness from coffee and the calming effects of CBD. The hope is the two will balance each other and you can say "good-bye" to caffeine jitters. Hempseed coffee is touted in the same manner.

One recent study shows some promise, citing that caffeine and cannabis compounds activate the same neurotransmitters.[44] There's no definitive science, though, to back up the claims that coffee and CBD are an ideal mix. There are no regulations, yet, either. But you will find a hefty price tag attached.

A cup of CBD coffee at a cafe can set you back ten dollars or more. A bag of CBD coffee beans for home brewing often costs upwards of twenty-five dollars.

Because the beans are typically coated with hemp or CBD oil, there is no guaranteed consistency or accuracy in dosing per cup. If the coffee house is brewing regular coffee and adding a CBD oil, there will be some more consistency in dosing, but as with any other combination, mixing CBD with coffee may alter the effects it has on your body. As happens when adding CBD oil to medicinal tea, heat may affect the potency and part of the oil may adhere to the cup.

Are hempseed oil and CBD coffees effective?

Potentially. Maybe? Effects will likely vary by person. For those who take full-spectrum CBD and find it makes them drowsy, dosing with caffeine-rich products known to increase alertness, like coffee, may offset the drowsiness.

Personally, I'm a huge fan of coffee. I often say it's my favorite "food group" (wink, wink). I'm also a bit of a self-professed coffee snob. I prefer to use a French press or pour-over method to brew my coffee. Many inexpensive coffee blends do not fare well with these brewing methods, as they are designed for drip brewers.

As such, most CBD-infused coffees have been a let-down in taste.

I have, however, found that taking CBD in the morning when I enjoy my daily brew does help negate the drowsy effect a bit. So, there may be some merit to that aspect. CBD affects everyone differently. Combining it with coffee may be a good solution for your specific needs.

Are hempseed oil and CBD coffees trendy? Absolutely!

If you're itching to try this trend, save a few dollars and try it at home. Brew your regular coffee in the morning, then add your CBD oil dose into your coffee, give it a stir, and enjoy your cup. Or, take your CBD oil in the morning and chase it with your favorite coffee brew.

If you find that the effects are desirable for you, you may want to splurge occasionally and enjoy a custom coffee-house brew.

 FRESH-BAKED TIP: You can add medicinal garden herbs and spices to your morning coffee. It can be a fun and flavorful way to add a bit more herbal power to your daily routine.

Turmeric, ginger, cinnamon, ashwagandha, nutmeg, mint, and cardamom are my favorites. You can add a little straight to your coffee grounds prior to brewing. Or you can mix in powdered herbs and spices directly into your cup after brewing for a stronger taste and effect.

CURATING ARTISAN COCKTAILS

It probably goes without saying, but cocktails are not an ideal, effective way to use medicinal herbs or CBD as a long-term, daily solution for your health and wellness goals.

Alcohol is a sedative. Full-spectrum CBD and many medicinal herbs can have a sedative effect. When used in abundance, you will likely have undesirable side effects.

Alcoholic beverages are also known to interfere with your sleep cycle. They impair your judgment. They may also interfere with medicines you're already taking. Always consult your doctor and pharmacist for potential interactions before imbibing any alcohol spirits.

Occasionally having a few sips of an herbal-infused cordial, however, or creating a custom cocktail using ingredients from your medicinal garden can be a fun treat. The key, naturally, is moderation!

Bartenders were temping us with botanical cocktails long before a happy hour was adopted into the bar trend scene. The mint julep is the official drink of the Kentucky Derby, companies like Ketel One offer botanical-infused spirits in their normal product line-up, and the Bloody Mary is a celebrated brunch staple.

Recently, with our global awakening of wellness, consumers have driven the demand for incorporating plant-based remedies and other health supplements into their cocktail hour.

It's speculative, at best, as to whether adding herbs or CBD oils to a cocktail actually offers any type of health or wellness enhancement. Truly little research exists. This is definitely an area where you should proceed with high caution, especially with CBD additives.

We have plenty of anecdotal evidence on many basic herbs, like mint, or spices, like cinnamon. These plants have been used for centuries to flavor alcoholic beverages. The FDA (fda.gov) lists these herbs and spices as safe for consumption.

We have still have no complete understanding of the effects CBD has on its own, let alone in combination with high quantities of alcohol. The FDA lists both alcohol and CBD as having potential side effects that include liver damage, reproductive toxicity, and a risk of sedation and drowsiness.

In a situation like this, I generally shy away from being the test subject at a local bar.

I'm also a fan of spending money wisely, and CBD-infused cocktails are double to triple the cost of a standard alcoholic beverage.

When it comes to medicinal gardening and alcohol, I have a different point of view. Alcohol preservation of plants is something we have a long history with. An occasional Bloody Mary or mimosa with brunch is a sweet treat.

This isn't to say there are no long-term effects of consuming alcohol, even in extreme moderation throughout your lifetime. Read the studies available (there are plenty) and decide for yourself if the benefits and drawbacks of occasional use are in line with your personal health and wellness goals.

If you do want to dabble with herb-infused alcohols, cordials are a potentially pleasant way to add a little botanical cocktail refreshment as an occasional treat. Herb-infused cordials are easy to create. You can enjoy a small glass after dinner, or add a few tablespoons to soda water, hot chocolate, coffee, tea, fruit juice, or other beverages to instantly create a botanical cocktail. You can also drizzle them on ice cream or desserts.

HERBAL CORDIALS—THIS IS JUST LIKE YOUR GRAND-MOTHER'S RECIPE!

To create an herb-infused cordial, you will need:

- vodka, rum, bourbon, brandy, or another pure (not flavored) alcohol of choice that is 80 proof or higher
- pure organic sugar
- purified water
- small saucepan
- fine mesh strainer
- 8-ounce mason jars
- fresh herbs of choice

Prior to creating cordials, be sure to read the "Important Canning Safety Tips" in Chapter 6. Then, you'll need to decide what flavor profile you want and what herbs may be best suited for your herbal cordial needs.

For example: If you're already using lemon balm regularly for its calming properties and you enjoy the flavor, creating a lemon balm-infused vodka cordial could be a good place to start.

Some of my favorite herbal cordial combinations are:

- rose petals + brandy
- mint + rum
- tarragon + bourbon

Use this chart for additional inspiration:

BASE ALCOHOL	PAIRS WELL WITH
Brandy	cinnamon, lemon peel, nutmeg, rose, vanilla
Bourbon	basil, cardamom, cilantro, mint, tarragon, vanilla
Gin	basil, cardamom, chamomile, coriander, cinnamon, ginger, lemon peel, lavender, lemongrass, orange peel, rosemary, sage, thyme
Rum	chamomile, ginger, lavender, lemon peel, lime peel, orange peel, mint, rosemary, tarragon
Tequila	cilantro, cinnamon, dill, lemon peel, lime peel, orange peel, rosemary
Vodka	Vodka is a great equalizer, meaning just about every spice, herb, fruit, or flower from your medicinal garden will pair well, as the flavors shine through this clear alcohol.
Whiskey	basil, cinnamon, coriander, ginger, ginseng, mint, orange peel, rosemary, sage, tarragon, vanilla

You will need three-fourths of a cup (six ounces) of fresh herbs (or rose petals) per eight-ounce mason jar you will be filling.

Each jar will need about one-third cup (three ounces) of simple syrup (created from sugar and water) and about two-thirds cup (six ounces) of alcohol.

The following recipe creates two eight-ounce jars of cordial or one sixteen-ounce jar.

ROSE PETAL BRANDY CORDIAL

Yield: 16 ounces (eight 2-ounce servings)

Ingredients:

2 cups organic sugar

1 cup purified water

1 1/3 cups of brandy (80 proof or higher)

1 1/2 cups wild rose petals

Rinse rose petals to remove any dirt or debris. Always use untreated organic rose petals from your medicinal garden.

Note: Do not use rose petals treated with pesticides, fertilizers, or other chemicals. You should *never* use roses from a florist or grocer. You may find untreated organic wild rose petals at your local farmer's market. Double-check with the farmer that they are indeed not treated with any chemicals, including chemical fertilizers.

Fill mason jar with rose petals (or, if using two eight-ounce mason jars, fill each with three-quarters cup of rose petals).

In a small saucepan, over a medium heat, add water and sugar. Stir continuously until sugar is fully dissolved into water. You should see no traces of sugar granules. This mix is referred to as "simple syrup." Remove from heat.

Cover rose petals in each jar, filling the jar one-third full of simple syrup (if you are using two eight-ounce jars, you'll use about one-third cup of simple syrup per jar).

You may find that you have a little simple syrup left over. Use it for sweetening medicinal teas and other beverages, or in your oatmeal or cereal in the morning. You can refrigerate it in a glass jar for use throughout the week.

Fill remainder of each mason jar with brandy. Gently stir contents of the jar with a spoon.

Seal jar(s) tightly. Store in a cool, dry, dark space for two weeks. Gently shake jar daily to encourage infusion of flavors.

After two weeks, open jar and use a fine mesh strainer to strain contents into a clean jar. Discard rose petals. Seal and label jar with contents and date.

Store in a cool, dry, dark space, and enjoy a small glass of your cordial as desired. Be sure to also adhere to the "Important Canning Safety" tips found in Chapter 6. Alcohol tinctures typically have a two-year shelf life when stored properly, but as you are only creating around eight servings per batch, they generally are used up much quicker!

Adding a little bit of honey or herb-infused honey to your whiskey and bourbon-based cordials can kick the flavor profile up a notch.

In the summertime, add two tablespoons of Rose Petal Brandy Cordial to eight ounces of soda water with a splash of fresh lemon juice for a refreshing cocktail twist.

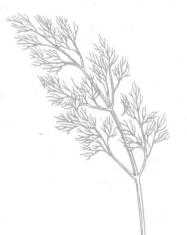

Creating Natural Bath, Beauty, and Home Remedies

SPLISH, SPLASH, TIME TO TAKE A CANNABINOID BATH!

Picture yourself slipping into a nice warm bath, tension leaving each muscle as comforting scents gently draw you into a lovely state of bliss. The hot bath does wonders for relaxing your body. Prolonged heat dilates blood vessels, promoting blood flow and allowing sore muscles to relax.

A hot bath mixed with the right botanicals can help de-stress, detox, and delight—completely rejuvenating your body, mind, and spirt.

CBD, touted for its anti-inflammatory properties and anti-anxiety effects, has become the popular new "it" ingredient for the seed-to-self movement, including bath and beauty products. If you already use oral cannabinoid for pain relief or muscle inflammation, considering CBD-infused products for topical relief is a natural progression.

Will you enjoy the calming and anti-anxiety effects of CBD in your bath time rituals? Likely not. In a hot bath, the cannabinoid will only be reacting with the surface of your skin and nearby cannabinoid receptors. For the full effects of CBD to be realized, it must be absorbed into your bloodstream.

That said, while CBD may not reach your bloodstream during a bath, it is absorbed by the skin, where the anti-inflammatory and pain-relieving aspects will come into play. A study published in 2016 concluded topical CBD application does have therapeutic potential for relief of arthritis pain and inflammation.[45] So you may enjoy some pain relief from your bath time CBD use.

We're all enchanted with new, natural products and ideas. CBD is a novelty right now and does have amazing potential in many applications. It's tempting to claim CBD is a "cure-all," but there's simply not enough research yet to back up these claims.

Ultimately, practicing nourishing self-care and providing much-needed relief to tired, sore muscles *is* beneficial. A hot bath is a wonderful treat, and adding CBD oil or hempseed oil to the mix is a lovely luxury that can amp up your results.

WHY DIY?

It's easy enough to purchase bath bomb, salts, or soaks, but there are plenty of solid reasons to strongly consider making your own.

First, it's super easy to do. Bath products take truly little time to create, and crafting them invests you fully in your self-care rituals.

More importantly, when you DIY, you have complete control over the amount and quality of ingredients. As we discussed in early chapters, not all CBD, hemp, and medicinal or aromatic botanicals are created equally. When you control the process from start to finish, you control the end results, ensuring you achieve the blissful experience you desire.

HEMPSEED OIL VERSUS CBD OIL

Long before CBD was isolated and extracted, full-spectrum hempseed oil popped into our bathing routines. It's been used to provide relief for several health concerns such as arthritis pain, PMS, menopause symptoms, and dry skin.

This power plant is well revered for its antioxidant and anti-inflammatory virtues. You'll find 10,000 years' worth of anecdotal and scientific data praising hemp's health and wellness properties. Industrial hemp was officially approved for use in cosmetic products in 2003.

Hempseed oil is derived from hempseeds. It has an abundance of essential fatty acids, making it a natural hair and skin soother, moisturizer, and softener. It's also chock full of omega acids, vitamins, protein, and minerals.

CBD oil is developed from plant flowers, making it a thicker substance called resin. It has a high content of CBD, which is why it has elevated levels of anti-oxidants and anti-inflammatory and pain-relieving properties. It does not have the same abundance of omega acids, vitamins, protein, and minerals that hempseed oil has.

As we discussed in Chapter 2, CBD oil is mixed with a carrier oil such as MCT or grapeseed. This carrier oil may have some beneficial hair and skin properties, like a high content of omega acids and proteins.

The question of using hempseed oil or CBD oil for bath and beauty products is easy if you're price conscious. As we've already learned, hempseed oil is considerably less expensive. You should be able to find hempseed oil for use with your bath and beauty DIY for around eight to ten dollars per thirty-two-ounce bottle.

Outside of price, if you're dealing with chronic pain or inflammatory diseases like eczema and psoriasis, CBD potentially offers more desirable results. Recent studies conclude that CBD oil inhibits inflammatory responses and pain.[46]

Note: If you're contending with chronic health issues and are new to cannabinoid products, it's prudent to consult with your current medical specialist, dermatologist, or other healthcare practitioners prior to using CBD skin products in combination with your current treatments. Regulations and data regarding marijuana, CBD, and related products is constantly developing.

If you're not contending with chronic pain or inflammatory diseases and just desire a natural hair and skin soother, moisturizer, and softener, hempseed oil is the clear choice.

In my personal experience, I've found that hempseed oil and CBD oil-infused bath bombs have both delivered rewarding results when used in my bath rituals.

I'm fortunately not dealing with any inflammatory skin issues or chronic pain conditions such as arthritis. I do manage lower back pain issues along with carpal tunnel syndrome, and I always find a hot bath brings much-needed relief.

Hempseed oil and CBD oil (due to its carrier oils) both have desirable skin soothing properties, and they do enhance my overall bath experience. As I don't usually need the boost in pain relief or anti-inflammatory properties CBD touts, I generally use hemp oil for its cost-saving benefits.

LET'S ALL BUILD A BATH BOMB!

Ready to create your own bath time nirvana? Bath bombs are a super fun way to begin your DIY self-care. In addition to being chock full of skin soothing ingredients, bath bombs deliver aromatic enhancements and colorful fizz to your hot bath.

You can find plenty of DIY kits at your local craft store or online. If you want to completely DIY your own, the basic tools and ingredients you need to get started are:

- **Bath bomb molds**—sphere molds designed specifically for bath bombs are available in plastic, metal, and silicone versions. Muffin tins and ice-cube trays also make excellent bath bomb molds.
- **Mixing bowls and whisk**—metal versions of each are desirable. Glass mixing bowls are a good option, too.
- **Epsom salts**—magnesium in Epsom salt also helps to relieve sore muscles.
- **Corn starch**—used to slow down the rate the bath bomb dissolves.
- **Citric acid**—reacts with baking soda to produces the "fizz" effect of the bath bomb. Alternatives to citric acid include lemon juice, cream of tartar, or apple vinegar.
- **Baking soda**—reacts with citric acid to produce "fizz" effect.
- **Essential oils**—optional ingredient. Used to include an aromatherapy component.

Of course, you'll also need your CBD or hempseed oil (or both!).

If you like colorful bath bombs, add a few drops of food coloring or mica color powder. I don't use these when creating my own, but it's a nice addition to have when you plan to use your bath bombs for gift giving.

A wealth of bath bomb recipes can be found with a simple Google search. If you'd like to get started right away, I've included my favorite personal recipe.

CLASSIC LAVENDER VANILLA BATH BOMB RECIPE

Yield: 2 average size (2-inch round) bath bombs

Ingredients:
1/2 cup baking soda
1/4 cup corn starch
1/4 cup citric acid
1/4 cup Epsom salt
1/2 teaspoon pure lavender
    essential oil
1/2 teaspoon pure vanilla essen-
    tial oil
1 teaspoon hempseed oil
1 teaspoon water
Optional—CBD oil

Note: If you decide you would like to add CBD oil to your bath bomb, you will first need to decide the number of milligrams you wish to have in your bath bomb. As we're reliant on anecdotal evidence, there is not an industry standard for amounts. CBD Bath Bombs currently sold in the marketplace generally contain 50–100 mg of CBD.

As with everything we've discussed pertaining to CBD dosing in this guide, start low! Try adding 50 mg of CBD per bath bomb on your initial run.

If you add CBD oil to the recipe, you may still need to add hempseed oil if you're adding under 5 ml of CBD oil (one teaspoon of hemp oil is about 5 ml) The oil helps bind the ingredients in your bath bomb, so it's an essential ingredient.

So, for example, assuming you wish to have 50 mg of CBD per bath bomb, you will need a total of 100 mg of CBD for the recipe, as this recipe yields two bath bombs. If your CBD oil tincture contains 25 mg of CBD per 1 ml dose, you will be adding 4 ml of CBD oil to the recipe.

You need 5 ml total (one teaspoon) of oil for the recipe. Therefore, you will want to add 1 ml of hempseed oil to ensure you have the full amount needed.

Once you have decided whether you wish to add CBD oil to your bath bomb and you have all your ingredients ready, to create, follow these quick and easy steps:

In a large mixing bowl, combine baking soda, corn starch, citric acid, and Epsom salt. Whisk gently until evenly mixed. Be sure to remove any lumps in mixture as you whisk.

In a small mixing bowl, combine essential oils, hempseed oil, and water. Whisk together until fully combined.

Add oil/water mixture to dry ingredients slowly, pouring in just a little at a time. Whisk continuously to combine. The mixture will fizz slightly. If it fizzes a lot, add smaller amounts of wet mixture. Continue until all ingredients are fully mixed.

The mixture should be sand-like at this stage and should easily stick together when pressed in your hand. If the mixture does not stick together in clumps when you squeeze it together in your hand, then add a little more water (a few drops at a time) until it easily clumps.

Line a countertop or cookie sheet with wax paper (or parchment paper).

Fill bath bomb molds completely with mixture, press mold together, and allow to dry for thirty minutes.

Gently release bath bomb from circular mold onto wax or parchment paper. Continue drying. I typically allow my bath bombs to dry overnight.

Store bath bombs in an airtight container in a cool, dry space. Use regularly to enjoy a soothing bath!

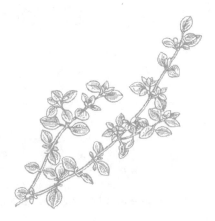

FRESH-BAKED TIP: Don't worry if your bath bomb crumbles when you release it from the mold. It happens sometimes due to all sorts of factors, including humidity. Just store the crumbed mixture in an airtight container and sprinkle it in your bath. You'll get the same benefits; you'll just be missing the pretty shape and prolonged fizz of the traditional bath bomb.

No time for a luxurious bath? You can still get the benefits of cannabinoid oil or hempseed oil in your shower by purchasing or creating your own soap.

DIY soap making is a little more time-consuming than fashioning bath bombs, but as you'll create a larger batch, your efforts will last longer. Again, you can find plenty of recipes with a simple internet search or purchase complete soap-making kits at your local craft-supply store.

ENHANCE YOUR BATH WITH AROMATHERAPY

In my favorite bath bomb recipe, I suggested using lavender and vanilla for their calming and relaxing properties. There's a wealth of aromatic options available to you when using essential oils.

Use this chart to create combinations to help you achieve your desired results. Feel free to experiment and come up with scent combinations on your own, too, until you find the perfect mix.

AROMATHERAPY BLEND	ESSENTAIL OIL 1		ESSENTAIL OIL 2
ENERGIZING MIX	1/2 teaspoon peppermint essential oil	+	1/2 teaspoon lemon essential oil
DAY BRIGHTENER	1/2 teaspoon orange essential oil	+	1/2 teaspoon vanilla essential oil

AROMATHERAPY BLEND (cont.)	ESSENTAIL OIL 1		ESSENTAIL OIL 2
UNDER-THE-WEATHER UPLIFTER	1/2 teaspoon lemon essential oil	+	1/2½ teaspoon eucalyptus essential oil
IMMUNITY BOOSTER	1/2 teaspoon oregano essential oil	+	1/2 teaspoon grapefruit essential oil
MUSCLE ACHE MIX	1/2 teaspoon lemongrass essential oil	+	1/2 teaspoon lavender essential oil
ANXIETY FIXER	1/2 teaspoon chamomile essential oil	+	1/2 teaspoon frankincense essential oil
SLEEP ENHANCER	1/2 teaspoon lavender essential oil	+	1/2 teaspoon chamomile essential oil
STRESS REDUCER	1/2 teaspoon clary sage essential oil	+	1/2 teaspoon lemon essential oil
MOOD FOR ROMANCE MIX	1/2 teaspoon sandalwood essential oil	+	1/2 teaspoon jasmine essential oil

For an extra kick, consider adding some of your medicinal garden produce to your bath bombs (or directly to your bath water). I love to add dried lavender flowers into my bath bomb mix or to sprinkle ground chamomile flowers directly into the bath water.

 FRESH-BAKED TIP: If you're interested in making DIY shower steamers, you can use the basic bath bomb recipe in this chapter. Just omit the hemp or CDB oils. For shower steamers, it's all about the aromatherapy!

MIX IT UP WITH BATH SALTS

Bath salts are a special treat like bath bombs, but even easier to create. Inexpensive and therapeutic, they are wonderful to have on hand and great for gift giving, too.

Commercial bath salts often contain chemicals that may irritate skin. By making bath salts at home, you'll save money and avoid unwanted additives.

To create, you will need:

- 1/2 cup of sea salt
- 1/2 cup of Epsom salt
- 20 drops of essential oil (in your favorite scent)
- small metal mixing bowl
- silicone spatula
- 4-ounce mason jars (the following recipe makes two 4-ounce jars)
- *Optional ingredient:* one-quarter cup of dried herbs (or *flowers*), finely chopped

I love to add dried lavender, chamomile, or mint to bath salts for their fragrance and color. They may, however, leave a residue on the bathtub after draining. It's easy enough to rinse off the residue, but not an aspect everyone appreciates.

To make bath salts: in a mixing bowl, add Epsom salt and sea salt. Stir to evenly distribute.

Optional: add dried herbs, stir to evenly distribute.

Add essential oil. (You can use twenty drops of one essential oil for a single scent or use ten drops from two different oils to create a mixed scent, like orange + vanilla). Stir rapidly to thoroughly mix oil with salts.

If any lumps form in the mixture, gently break them up using the edge of the spatula.

Pour salts into jars. Seal and store in a cool, dry space. Use as needed.

FRESH-BAKED TIP: Having issues with dry skin? After adding your homemade bath salts to your bath, pour one cup of apple cider vinegar into your bath water. Apple cider vinegar is a natural skin soother that also helps unclog pores and exfoliate skin.

After your bath, you may have a trace of apple cider vinegar scent on your skin. If this bothers you, simply rinse off in the shower for a minute after your bath.

MANE ATTRACTION—MEDICINAL HAIR TEAS

Medicinal garden teas are not just for drinking, they are also a powerful tonic for your hair. Botanicals are commonly used in commercial hair products for their benefits and aromas. Why not create your own experience at home with your medicinal garden plants?

Whether you have trouble with dandruff or just want some extra shine, there's a hair tea that may be a great help in supporting your needs.

To create medicinal hair teas, use one-half cup of fresh herbs per two cups of water.

If you have short to medium length hair, two cups of hair tea are plenty. If you have long hair, you may want to brew a total of four cups.

First, using a tea kettle (or small saucepan), bring water to a boil. Remove from heat. Add fresh herbs to boiling water. Steep for one hour.

After one hour, strain herbs from water and discard herbs. Pour hair tea into a shatter-proof cup or any other vessel that will be safe to use in your bathroom or shower.

Wash and rinse hair per your normal routine, but skip the use of your conditioner.

After washing your hair, slowly pour hair tea over hair and scalp, gently massaging it in with your fingertips.

Note: As with any hair product, avoid contact with your eyes and other sensitive body parts. If it gets in or near your eyes, flush with water immediately.

After rinsing your hair with hair tea, leave the tea residue in your hair—do not rinse it out with water. If you're showering, rather than washing your hair, you will want to rinse your body to remove any tea residue.

Towel dry hair. If preferred, you may spray your hair with a leave-in conditioner or use a hair oil after drying. Proceed to style your hair as you normally would.

Hair teas may be used once per week (or more often), depending upon your personal preferences and needs. You should notice subtle effects immediately after your first use of a hair tea. Over time, the effects tend to have a cumulative effect. Using chamomile hair tea on blond hair, for example, should help brighten the hair and add a little shine after the first use. Over time, you may notice some lightening of the hair color. If you feel you've reached an optimal stage for your hair color and brightness, discontinue the hair tea use from your routine for a while, and then add it back in when you feel your hair needs some extra pep.

You may also choose to switch hair teas. If you find that your blond hair is lightening from regular chamomile tea use, but all you want is some shine to your hair, stop using the chamomile hair tea in your routine and brew some lavender hair tea instead.

Use this guide to help you determine the best hair tea(s) for your hair needs:

- **Blond hair**—brew chamomile hair tea
- **Brown hair**—brew rosemary hair tea
- **Dark hair**—brew sage hair tea
- **Red hair**—brew calendula flower hair tea
- **Oily hair**—brew lemongrass hair tea OR brew thyme hair tea
- **Dandruff**—brew bay leaf hair tea
- **Split ends**—brew catnip hair tea
- **To add shine to any color hair**—brew lavender hair tea OR brew basil hair tea

There's no tried-and-true solution for gray hair, but you may find that chamomile hair tea (for light gray or white hair) or sage hair tea (for dark gray hair) have desirable effects in helping to even out hair tones. Lavender hair tea is a lovely option for all shades of gray hair, as it will add shine and luster.

For each shampoo session, use only one hair tea. If you have multiple hair needs, alternate use of hair teas throughout the week.

For example: If you have blond hair and dandruff issues, use a chamomile hair tea the first time you wash your hair during the week and a bay leaf hair tea the next time you wash your hair that week.

Use apple cider vinegar for hair as a bonus boost, especially when dandruff is one of your common hair issues. Once per week, prior to using your hair tea, rinse hair with one cup of apple cider vinegar first.

Looking for an all-natural conditioner to pamper your locks a little more? A combination of hempseed oil and rose water is a refreshing treat for every hair type.

To create a rose water hempseed oil conditioner use:

- 1/2 cup of rose water (see recipe in Chapter 8)
- 1/4 cup of hempseed oil

Whisk rose water and hempseed oil together.

After shampooing your hair, massage rose water hempseed oil conditioner into hair and scalp. Continue massaging hair, using your fingertips to ensure all hair strands are coated.

Leave rose water hempseed oil conditioner on for five minutes and then rinse out. If you have extremely dry hair, don't rinse the mixture out. Leave it in for extra conditioning.

Dry and style hair per your normal routine.

 FRESH-BAKED TIP: Medicinal hair teas can also be used as an herbal facial treatment.

- Rose petals hydrate dry skin.
- Chamomile and lavender are skin soothers.
- Peppermint can help detox and refresh.
- Parsley and lemongrass are natural astringents, good for balancing oily skin.
- Rosemary helps brighten all skin types.

Note: Always be mindful of allergies and test a small patch of your skin before applying a full facial. Also be sure to avoid your eye area, nose, and mouth.

To create an herbal tea facial experience, brew hair tea per normal. After herbs are strained from the tea, fully moisten two washcloths with tea.

Place washcloths on a clean plate. Microwave for ten seconds or until cloths are warm to the touch. Cloths should be warm, not hot. If too hot, allow to cool down a bit first before using.

Lie back on a reclining chair, couch, or another comfortable spot where you can lean back slightly. Arrange cloths on face and leave on for five minutes for a refreshing, relaxing facial.

For herbs I know I do well with and have no allergies to, I tent the cloth over my mouth and nose for a few minutes for a little extra aromatic steam therapy experience. Use your discretion.

If you have extra herbal tea left over, save it in a sealed container in the refrigerator for up to three days for use in your bath water. When you draw your bath, simply pour the leftover herbal tea in.

TIME FOR THE AFTER-BATH!

As we already touched on, hempseed oil is found in a lot of modern beauty products including skin-care creams. It's a lovely moisturizer for all skin types.

A hempseed-oil body butter or moisturizing cream is not the same as a CBD-infused cream or salve. You may find CBD and hempseed oil in the same product. In this instance, the hempseed oil is typically acting as a carrier agent for the CBD oil.

The biggest difference between the two when it comes to external care is their intent:

- **CBD-infused topicals** (like creams and salves) are primarily intended for use as a pain reliever for muscle aches, arthritis, or skin irritations.
- **Hempseed oil topicals** (like body butters and creams) are designed to help moisturize and aid in overall skin health.

CBD topicals come with a hefty price tag attached, too. Hempseed oil topicals are generally far less expensive, unless additional ingredients like an anti-aging compound are added to it.

If you want to have a little DIY fun, creating hempseed-oil body butter is a great way to start. This luxurious moisturizer not only smells great, it hydrates and pampers your skin.

In my experience, hempseed-oil body butter leaves your skin silky smooth and soft to the touch. During a time when hand-sanitizers are stripping oils from our skin, I've been extra glad to have some sumptuous body butter on hand.

 FRESH-BAKED TIP: Have trouble with ragged cuticles? Try my favorite cuticle fix:

Mix one teaspoon of hempseed oil with one teaspoon of vitamin E oil. Every night before bedtime, rub a little bit of this oil mixture into your cuticles and surrounding skin and nail bed.

As I tend to impromptu spot-garden when I'm outside without the aid of garden gloves—aka when I see a weed I pull it, or when I see a plant that needs tending I tend to it—my cuticles suffer. This oil mix works wonders. Each night when needed I rub some in, and in the morning my dry, ragged skin is well on its way to repair.

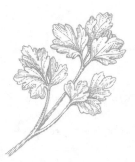

HEMPSEED-OIL BODY BUTTER

Yield: 8 ounces (I generally use two 4-ounce mason jars so I can keep one in the bathroom and one near the kitchen sink for use after washing dishes or cleaning up from garden work.)

Ingredients:

1/2 cup shea butter
1/4 cup hempseed oil
1/2 teaspoon of vitamin E oil
small saucepan
silicon spatula
hand mixer
medium-size metal (or glass)
*   mixing bowl*
Optional: a few drops of essen-
*   tial oil in your favorite scent*

In a small saucepan, over a low heat, melt shea butter, stirring constantly. Once shea butter is fully melted, remove from heat.

Pour shea butter into mixing bowl. Stir in hempseed oil. Mix until thoroughly combined.

Place bowl in refrigerator for five minutes (or until the shea butter mixture begins to resolidify). It will be soft to the touch—do not fully reharden the mix.

Remove bowl from refrigerator. Add vitamin E oil and (optionally) add essential oil drops.

Using a hand mixer, mix on low speed until oils are incorporated. Use spatula to scrape down sides of bowl.

Switch mixer speed to high and whip body butter for ten minutes (or until mixture is airy and doubles in size).

Transfer hempseed-oil body butter to jars.

Seal jars and use regularly. This body butter will generally have a shelf life of six months, but you'll probably use it up within one to two months.

Use fingers to scoop a small amount of body butter and rub into hands, arms, elbows, knees, or anywhere you could use some skin TLC.

Note: After making hempseed body butter, always first test a small amount of body butter on a small patch of skin to ensure you experience no unwanted side effects like allergic reactions or blemishes due to clogged pores (especially if using as a face cream).

Hempseed-oil body butter is generally too heavy for use as a facial moisturizer. For those with dry to normal skin, however, it may be a lovely occasional night cream moisturizer to try.

CAN YOU ADD CBD OIL TO YOUR HEMPSEED-OIL BODY BUTTER?

Yes.

Will it be effective for anxiety reduction or as a muscle relaxant? Just as we discussed in the "Let's All Build a Bath Bomb!" section, likely not.

If you're using CBD creams for their anti-inflammatory properties to add with conditions like arthritis, you may see some minor benefit from adding CBD oil to your hempseed-oil body butter.

If you want to try, you can swap out the vitamin E oil in the hempseed-oil body butter recipe for half teaspoon of CBD oil. You may find that it works as effectively for you as some commercial CBD creams or salves that are available. You may not. However, keep in mind the expense may outweigh the benefit here.

For quick reference, a 15 ml bottle of CBD contains approximately three teaspoons. If the 15 ml bottle contains 200 mg of CBD, then each half teaspoon serving will contain about 33 mg of CBD.

A standard commercial CBD cream typically contains about 400–500 mg of CBD per bottle. To achieve that level in your body butter recipe, you would typically have to use a full 15 ml bottle of CBD containing 500 mg per bottle and reduce the amount of hempseed oil in the recipe (which will alter the consistency and intent of the hemp body butter as a skin softening agent). It will also up the cost of producing your hempseed body butter dramatically.

If your wellness goals do not include managing chronic pain like arthritis or an inflammatory skin condition like eczema, a CBD-infused topical will offer little benefit. A better product to use for managing chronic pain like arthritis or occasional muscles aches is a CBD salve. You can purchase a variety of CBD-infused salves and creams designed specifically for this purpose, or you can simply make your own.

DIY CBD OIL SALVE

As we discussed in Chapter 5, a great product to add to your natural first aid kit is a CBD-infused salve. They are particularly handy to have when you're hiking or participating in other strenuous activities like kayaking, working out, or just partaking in a friendly round of volleyball with your friends on a beach vacation. As you're often energized and involved in the moment, you can sometimes overdo things a bit and wind up with sore muscles.

CBD's anti-inflammatory properties may help alleviate some of the pain associated with muscle strain when taken orally, but also when applied directly to the skin. Combining CBD with essential oils like turmeric, peppermint, and eucalyptus will help with the effectiveness of your salve and also give it a great scent.

As a side note, you can make this salve without CDB oil, too. Essential oils on their own can often provide the right amount of relief.

This recipe yields about two ounces of salve. Rather than creating a full two-ounce batch of CBD oil salve, my advice is to create a half batch of CBD oil salve, and a half batch of salve without the CBD oil. This way you will be able to try the salve with and without CBD to see if there's any noticeable difference for you.

To create my CBD oil salve you will need:

- 2 tablespoons coconut oil
- 2 tablespoons hempseed oil
- 1 tablespoon beeswax (I like to use beeswax pellets, because they are easy to measure, they melt well, and you can find them at most craft/ hobby stores)
- 5 drops of peppermint essential oil
- 5 drops turmeric essential oil
- 5 drops of eucalyptus essential oil
- CBD oil
- double boiler
- silicone spatula
- 4-ounce mason jars

Note: if you prefer a different essential oil, such as camphor essential oil or winter-green essential oil (both also known for aiding with muscle relief), you may substitute them for any of the essential oils I've suggested.

Deciding how many milligrams of CBD to add to your salve can be a little tricky at first, especially if you have never tried a CBD salve before. If you have tried a salve and enjoyed the results, you can simply refer to the canister to find out how many milligrams of CBD are present in the one you've used. If you haven't, it may mean some trial and error initially to determine the perfect amount for your particular needs.

A CBD salve doesn't necessarily have a set amount per dose, as the quantity you use may vary by need. Some days you may need just a dab to deal with a bit of neck strain from sitting at your computer too long. Other times you will need a big scoop of salve to help ease hamstring pain after hiking.

Commercial CBD salves are not always consistent with dosage formulation. Some contain only trace amounts of CBD (around 25 mg per ounce of salve) and others an excessive amount (upward of 600 mg of CBD or more per ounce of salve). The average seems to land somewhere around 100–200 mg of CBD per ounce of salve.

As I wholeheartedly believe in the notion of starting with lower doses of CBD, I suggest beginning with adding a 100 mg dose of CBD oil per ounce, maximum. If you will be adding CBD to the entire recipe, this means you will need 200 mg of CBD. If your 15 ml vial of CBD oil contains 400 mg of CBD, this means you will be adding 7.5 ml of CBD oil. (Refer to the charts in Chapter 2 and Chapter 7 to help you calculate your CBD measurements for this recipe.)

To begin making your CBD oil salve, set up your double boiler and place it on the stove over a medium heat.

Note: if you don't have a double boiler, you can find plenty of instructions online on how to create a mock double boiler using a saucepan and a glass or stainless steel mixing bowl.

Add beeswax to top pan of the double boiler. Heat until beeswax is fully melted, stirring occasionally.

Once beeswax is fully melted, add coconut oil and hemp oil. Stir until wax and oils are fully combined. Remove from heat and allow to cool for five minutes.

Add essential oils and stir until oils are fully incorporated into mixture.

If you are splitting the recipe: at this stage, evenly divide the mixture between two mason jars. Add a 100 mg dose of CBD oil to one of the mason jars, mix well to ensure the oil is evenly distributed throughout the mixture. Be sure to mark the outside of the jar with a permanent marker, sticker, or some type of label to help you remember which jar contains CBD.

If you are not splitting the recipe, pour entire mixture into one mason jar. Add a 200 mg dose of CBD oil to the jar. Mix well to ensure the oil is evenly distributed throughout the entire mixture.

Leave jar(s), with the lid off, to cool for about six hours. I generally make this salve at night and allow it to cool and resolidify overnight.

Once salve has solidified, seal with lid and store in a cool, dark spot such as a bathroom medicine cabinet. Use as needed for sore muscle pain relief. Salve will generally store well for six to nine months before ingredients begin to degrade, loose their effectiveness, or separate.

To use, scoop out a bit of the salve and rub into the affected area. It's best to test out on a small spot of skin first, such as the top of your wrist, to ensure the salve does not aggravate your skin and that you do not have any allergic reactions to the ingredients. Do note that this salve is for external use *only*, and it is best to avoid any sensitive skin areas, including all areas of your face. If you experience any allergic reaction, wash salve off immediately. If the reaction is severe, seek medical attention immediately.

If you're testing to see how well the CBD oil salve works versus the salve without CBD oil, try alternating applications when you find a need for use. Then make note of any differences to help you to decide whether you will continue adding CBD oil to your salve or if the essential oil mix suits your needs without the addition of CBD.

If you find that the CBD oil version works best but still doesn't quite help enough, you can begin to up the dosage of CBD milligrams per ounce for your next batch. Continue adding a little at a time with each new batch until you find your optimum formula.

HEMPSEED-OIL SUGAR SCRUB

Sugar scrubs are a brilliant way to utilize the skin nourishing features of hempseed oil. This indulgent scrub promotes healthy skin through gentle exfoliation and moisturizing.

It's ridiculously easy and inexpensive to create a luxurious hempseed oil sugar scrub, and your skin will totally thank you for it!

There are two types of sugar I highly recommend for use when creating sugar scrubs:

1. Dark brown sugar—for all-purpose sugar scrubs
2. Turbinado sugar (raw sugar)—for trouble spots like legs, feet, and elbows

All you need to create a hempseed oil sugar scrub is hempseed oil and sugar. I love to add in skin-care friendly plants from my medicinal garden, too, like dried lavender, dried rose petals, or dried mint leaves. You can also pop in a few drops of essentials oils for an aromatherapy component.

My favorite all-purpose sugar scrub blend is a combination of dark brown sugar, hempseed oil, and lemon balm.

LEMON BALM HEMPSEED-OIL SUGAR SCRUB

Ingredients:
2 cups dark brown sugar
1/2 cup hempseed oil
1/4 cup dried lemon balm leaves,
*   ground fine*
8-ounce wide mouth mason jar

In a small mixing bowl, add hempseed oil, sugar, and lemon balm. Mix thoroughly until all ingredients are fully incorporated and evenly distributed.

Pour mixture into mason jar, seal, and store near your sink or shower for regular use. This scrub will generally stay fresh for one to two months.

If you have leftover scrub after filling your mason jar, use it to pamper yourself for a DIY job well done!

CBD AND ORAL HEALTH—IS THAT A THING?

We've covered all your skin surfaces and hair rituals, now it's time to address one of your best beauty assets—your smile!

My mother always encouraged good dental habits in our household. She placed as much importance on dental care as she did every other aspect of good hygiene and health. The Office of Disease Prevention and Health Promotion (ODPHP) agrees, stating clearly "The health of the teeth, the mouth, and the surrounding craniofacial (skull and face) structures is central to a person's overall health and well-being."[47]

Some oral health professionals and researchers, including Dr. Heather Kunen, DDS, MS, cofounder of Beam Street (beam-st.com), believe CBD may have an important place in the oral health care arena.

"CBD is known to reduce inflammation throughout the human body, and it has the same effect on our oral tissues," says Dr. Kunen. "I'm excited to think about how we may be able to use it for pain relief, as an anti-inflammatory, and as an analgesic in dental care."

There are pharmaceutical companies and scientists currently exploring cannabis oral care solutions, but more research needs to be done. Periodontal disease (infections and inflammation of the gums and bone surrounding teeth) affects over 47 percent of adults aged 30 years and older.[48] Exploring the anti-inflammatory and antibacterial properties of cannabis compounds like CBD makes sense.

A preliminary study shows that cannabinoids "have the potential to be used as an effective antibacterial agent against dental plaque-associated bacteria."[49]

Dr. Kunen also suggests a benefit to CBD use may also be its ability to help reduce anxiety (which, we all know, can be extremely helpful in a dental setting for many!). As we already explored in Chapter 2, several studies support CBD's anti-anxiety properties.

"Hopefully, over time the stigma dissipates, as people become more educated and informed about cannabis," says Dr. Kunen. "Could be in the near future that we carry dental products with CBD or other cannabis plant compounds."

Dr. Kunen does warn that CBD oil may have one adverse dental effect—causing a patient to have dry mouth. This can lead to oral tissue discomfort. To prevent, it's particularly important for patients to stay well hydrated when consuming CBD in any form.

You can stay up to date on the latest oral care health information, including the role of cannabis in oral health, by visiting the American Dental Association website (ada.org). In the future, if you opt to use a CBD-infused oral care product, do consult your dental care professional first, and also be mindful of looking for all the important indicators for a quality product that we reviewed in Chapters 2 and 3.

 FRESH-BAKED TIP: Did you know that some of the herbs from your medicinal garden can help freshen your breath?

Parsley is the star garnish for its ability to freshen breath. Chew it after your meal, and you can keep the dinner conversation going without bad breath interfering.

Drinking dill tea or chewing on dill seeds works well, too. Cardamom seeds work in the same way, though they can be a bit too spicy for some people.

Of course, mint is a powerhouse when it comes to disguising bad smells and freshening breath. Nip off a few leaves from your plant and chew them to make your breath minty fresh.

FRAGRANT HERBS FOR YOUR HOME

From using pressed leaves or flowers for decoupage to boiling plants for natural dyes for linens, herbs (and spices) have been enhancing home décor for centuries.

Bundles of dried herbs make lovely long-lasting floral arrangements, especially lavender. Dried seed pods and dried flowers can be used to decorate picture frames or wreaths. A few sprigs of rosemary and a bit of twine can be fashioned into a rustic napkin holder for holiday gatherings.

You'll find endless ways to use your excess herbs and plant matter.

If we approach it from a medicinal herb viewpoint, the key to your overall health, wellness, and happiness in your home is aromatherapy.

Herbs and spices house the power to change your environment through your sense of sight and smell. Uplifting scents like lemon verbena and peppermint can lighten your mood instantly. A bowl of potpourri makes a beautiful décor statement.

Using medicinal plants in your home can also help detox your space, improving air quality by eliminating the need for chemical-heavy air fresheners. If you grow some of your medicinal plants indoors, it can also have a positive effect on the air clarity in your home, as plants are natural air filters.

For the best effect, try to spread your medicinal container garden plants throughout your home. Some, like rosemary and mint, will naturally lightly scent the air in a room as they grow. Others provide better aromas after they are dried, or their essential oils are extracted for use in air fresheners, candles, and potpourri.

Making potpourri is one of the fastest ways to add subtle, long-lasting scent to any room. For a quick mix use:

- 1/2 cup dried flowers (or flower petals)
- 1/2 cup dried herb leaves
- 1 tablespoon of dried citrus rind or dried spices (like cinnamon sticks, bay leaves, or coriander seeds)

Gently mix these ingredients together and place in a potpourri jar. You can find jars at your local craft store or online.

You can also create a DIY potpourri jar with a mason jar, cheesecloth, and a length of twine or ribbon. Place the potpourri in the jar. Cover the top of the jar with a square of cheesecloth that overlaps the opening of the jar. Secure the cheesecloth to the top of the jar with twine or ribbon.

The cheesecloth helps release the scent slowly. You can opt to leave the jar wide open; the potpourri will just have a shorter shelf life (and may collect dust more easily).

Always use dried plant matter. Fresh plant matter may be laid out in a room to help scent it temporarily, but you will find that it molds and/or rots quickly when clumped together.

Some of my favorite potpourri combinations are:

- rose petals + chamomile flowers + cinnamon sticks
- rose petals + lemongrass + clove
- lavender flowers + bay leaves + coriander
- lavender flowers + lemon verbena + lemon peel
- chamomile flowers + mint leaves + orange peel

If you happen to have a pine tree on your property, a combination of pine branches, cinnamon sticks, and dried nutmeg is a delightful scent for the winter holidays.

Potpourri can easily be enhanced with other items like pinecones, pine branches, seed pods, star anise, and dried fruit to enhance scent and visual appeal.

To strengthen or revive your potpourri scents, add a few drops of essential oils to the mix. If you want to fill your entire home with rich aromatics, pour your potpourri into a crockpot filled with water. Leave the lid off and set the crockpot too low.

Allow potpourri to simmer in crockpot for several hours. As the water warms, the delightful scents will be released to perfume your home.

Afterward, drain the water and discard or compost the potpourri plant materials.

 FRESH-BAKED TIP: Create small batches of potpourri to scent your closet and drawers. Commonly referred to as "sachets," this practice was once wildly popular and used to help clothing from getting too musty. It's still enjoyed today for its pleasing effects.

Use small sachet bags or use your medicinal tea bags to contain the potpourri for your small spaces.

My favorite closet and dresser drawer scent combinations are:

- cinnamon + cloves + orange peel
- lavender + mint
- rosemary + thyme
- sage + peppermint
- lavender + rose petals

IS THERE ANY ADVANTAGE TO ADDING CBD TO HOME PRODUCTS LIKE POTPOURRI?

This may sound like a silly question to some, but with CBD popping up in everything from workout gear to pillows, it's a valid question to ask.

The answer—no, not really. Not that we know of.

There's currently no reason to believe or science that supports the need for CBD compounds in home goods like blankets, potpourri, or candles. Essential oils from medicinal herbs and spices in candles, on the other hand, can enhance a home with wonderful aromas that may induce relaxing, uplifting, or calming feelings.

GET LIT WITH DIY HERBAL SOY CANDLES

I'm someone who absolutely adores using candles in my home. I've got plenty of them stashed around here with different scents for different moods.

When I'm cleaning, I love to light soy candles with lemony scents like lemon verbena, lemongrass, and lemon balm. They energize my mood while delivering a fresh, crisp, clean scent to each area I'm working on.

Rosemary, cinnamon, and peppermint are my go-tos for times when I'm writing. Whether they increase my focus or not (an effect all three plants are known for), they sure smell terrific and help brighten my space.

Sage, vanilla, and thyme are some of my favorite evening scents. I find them soothing and relaxing.

Sometimes I purchase candles or receive them as gifts, but I also enjoy making them. Occasionally I DIY my essential oils using the slow-cooker method (see recipe in Chapter 6), but most often I have plenty of pure essential oils on-hand that I've purchased for my DIY bath products, air fresheners, or potpourri refreshing.

Soy wax and wicks can be found at your local craft store. If you plan to make candles regularly, you may also want to consider purchasing a wax warmer and other specialty items like a natural soy candle making kit.

To create soy candles, you will need:

- mason jars (I prefer wide mouth jars)
- soy wax for container candles (not the wax for molded candles—the container should specify type)
- wicks for candles that have been tabbed and primed (appropriate for size of jar, again the packaging will help you identify proper sizes)
- wick tabs for attaching wick to bottom of jar
- essential oils
- melting pot (small slow cookers work well, or you can use a saucepan in a pinch)
- large glass measuring cup with pouring spout
- silicone spatula
- food/candy thermometer

Wide mouth mason jars work well as your candle holder, but you may use other containers like a ceramic vessel. You'll need to choose a clean, heat-resistant, nonflammable container that won't shatter when the heat from a candle flame hits it.

Decide how many candles you want to make. One pound of soy wax will make three eight-ounce mason jar candles (*with some wax left over*). Or it will fill one sixteen-ounce mason jar and one eight-ounce mason jar (*with some wax left over*).

Begin the candle-making process by melting your soy wax. If you are using a slow cooker, use the warm setting. If you are using a saucepan, you'll want to warm the wax on an exceptionally low heat, simmering it until melted. The key is low heat, slow melt.

Using wick tabs, attach wicks for candles to the bottoms of the jars you will be using for your candles. (Follow manufacturer's instructions on package.)

Secure the wick so that it will stand upright while you are pouring the candle wax. A tried-and-true method is to wrap the top of the wick around a pencil and tie it. I use a wood skewer for mine. You can also buy wick sticks at your craft store for this purpose.

When wax is fully melted and reaches at least 190 degrees Fahrenheit, remove from heat. Pour wax into measuring cup with pouring spout.

Add one ounce of essential oils per one pound of soy wax used. Stir oil into the wax until oil and wax are thoroughly combined.

Slowly pour the wax into your candle jar. Wax should be poured to the side of the wick, not over it. Fill jar, leaving a small headspace near the rim so that wax will not spill over the jar when you first begin to burn the candle.

Allow the candle to cool overnight. When cooled, trim wick to about a quarter inch. Seal the jar and let it cure for two weeks. This allows the scent to develop as it cures.

After two weeks, when the curing period is over, light the candle and enjoy the fresh aromatics throughout your home.

10. GET ENLIGHTENED
Celebrating Your New Lifestyle and Discovering Additional Resources

This morning, I started my day by clipping fresh herbs from my garden.

Cilantro and sage are left to dry on racks to be stored for use later. Basil and garlic (from last year's harvest) quickly become pesto for tonight's dinner.

Mint is chopped and made into ice cubes for glasses of iced tea throughout the week. Lemon verbena is set aside for a medicinal tea, which I'll pair with the mint-infused honey I created last month.

I pop a dash of ginger in my coffee as I take out cinnamon, turmeric, and hemp hearts for my oatmeal.

Next, I pour a glass of water and invite my CBD capsule into my daily rituals before tidying up the kitchen and sitting down for a quick breakfast break.

After breakfast, I'll light a lemongrass soy candle to freshen my home as I begin my daily chores.

If my morning sounds serene and idyllic—it is.

It's not always, of course, since, well, life happens! But, as often as possible, I stick to my routine because it works well and starts my day off on a healthy and meditative note. This prepares me for all of life's rollercoaster moves in the day ahead.

I hope it sounds like something you can easily incorporate a step at a time into your lifestyle, too, because—it is.

I'd like to profess that I got here overnight. I didn't. It takes work, dedication to self-care, time, and plenty of patience. It takes being kind to yourself and making an effort to consistently address all your needs.

This is often easier said than done, I totally understand that. It would be wonderful if I could share that I'm 100 percent where I want to be health-wise. Nope, I'm constantly a work in progress.

What I can share with certainty is that if you place your health and wellness as a high priority, you can make positive strides toward improving your life. Self-care is often undervalued, and we sometimes mistake it for selfishness. What better gift can you give to the world, though, than being your best you?

While it may be self-centric, it's not selfish to place your healthcare high on your daily list of to-dos. When you're in a good space mentally, emotionally, spiritually, and physically, you're in a much better position to support the loved ones in your life and to deal with all the ups and downs in your world, and the world at-large.

My day is idyllic in another way, too. Every day I feel healthy.

I'm not cured, and I still have chronic health issues like carpal tunnel syndrome and Hashimoto's thyroiditis. My eyes are aging—I just had to get bifocals. I weigh more than I'd like to.

Despite all this, I feel healthy.

I'm well rested, energetic, and focused with clarity of mind. Even though I'm in premenopause with low estrogen levels, my mood is balanced. My chronic issues are still here, but I'm better able to manage them with the aid of CBD and medicinal plants. For whatever crops up, from sunburn to occasional digestive woes, I have natural solutions on hand.

If you feel healthy and your overall wellness is tended to, there's no better feeling. As the notion goes—the person who has health has hope. And the person who has hope has the whole shebang!

My day is filled with flavor, my meals are lively. Nothing compares to the taste of a fresh herb or spice that you nurtured, harvested, and prepared yourself.

Hopefully, after reading this guide, you've found that whether you work at home, work outside the home, travel regularly, are a full-time caretaker, or are juggling a variety of roles (as most of us do), hemp, CBD, and medicinal gardening are easy to seamlessly incorporate into your daily routines in a variety of ways.

My morning and my day also include a few natural supplements and medicinal garden plants that are not included in this guide. Generally, this is because they are not common to the United States—for example, Triphala, a traditional Ayurvedic formula comprised of three fruits: amalaki, bibhitaki, and haritaki. Or it may be because they are more advanced medicinal plants that are either foraged, an acquired taste, and/or not commonly found in the average garden.

Starting in a familiar space with familiar medicinal plants helps you more easily form habits and enjoy the experience, and ensures you have a modicum of success that will inspire and empower you to continue integrating natural remedies into your lifestyle.

You have all the basics you need now to move forward on your journey.

As your next step, consider hiring a local foraging expert to take a walk around your property to discover all the wild edibles in your backyard. Discuss additional medicinal plants that might fit in well with your landscape and terrain.

Begin exploring additional medicinal plants that help with health issues, like St. John's Wort for easing stress and symptoms of depression, or valerian as a sleep aid. When you're ready for the next level, you'll find plenty of resources available, including herbalist classes, advanced books, and naturalist clubs you can join.

Keep in mind, new cannabis technologies and innovations in the United States will continue to develop, too. You'll want to stay tuned in for the exciting new chapters in our medicinal plant history as they unfold.

Be sure to check out the following resource section for some starting points to help you walk the next path.

I'm grateful you opted to begin your journey with me, and I hope that you've found plenty of ways to enhance and support your holistic wellness needs. I wish you good health and a lifetime full of joy as you continue to explore new trails.

Stay wild and stay well!

Hemp, CBD, and Medicinal Garden Resources

Stay up to date with the newest developments in consumer cannabis laws and regulations, find educational opportunities, and further your hemp, CBD, and medicinal garden journey with these resources:

American Botanical Council (abc.herbalgram.org)—provides education to promote the responsible use of herbal medicine

American Herbal Pharmacopoeia (herbal-ahp.org)—promotes responsible use of herbal medicines and herbal medicine safety

Earth Law Center (earthlawcenter.org)—nonprofit established to transform the law to protect nature

Hemp Industries Association (thehia.org)—nonprofit association working to change regulations and policies prohibiting the use of hemp for commercial purposes

Hemp Industry Daily (hempindustrydaily.com)—covers current financial, legal, and business news for the hemp industry

Herb Research Foundation (herbs.org)—current news and education on herbs and other natural products for health and natural healing

Leafly (leafly.com)—detailed information on cannabis strains, trends, terpenes, and products

Millia Magazine (milliamagazine.com)—magazine focused on cannabis and the cannabis cultural perspectives

Ministry of Hemp (ministryofhemp.com)—covers new trends and developments in the hemp industry

National Association of State Departments of Agriculture (NASDA) (nasda.org)—nonpartisan, nonprofit association that represents the elected and appointed commissioners, secretaries, and directors of the departments of agriculture in all fifty states and four U.S. territories

National Hemp Association (nationalhempassociation.org)—nonprofit organization dedicated to the growth and development of the industrial hemp industry

NORML (norml.org)—organization established to serve as an advocate for cannabis consumers

The Herbal Academy (herbalacademy.com)—provides herbal education courses, workshops, and resources

United Plant Savers Medicinal Plant Conservation (unitedplantsavers.org)—research, education, and conservation of native medicinal plants and their habitats

Recipe and Instruction Index

ABOUT THE AUTHOR

 BARB WEBB is a freelance writer, author, blogger, and sustainable living expert. When she's not chasing chickens around the farm or engaging in mock-Jedi battles with her sons, she's writing about homesteading and artisan culture.

Born under the earth sign Taurus, Barb arrived in the world ready to start nurturing, digging, and planting! She believes the universe is an excellent guide if we simply open our minds and hearts to listen.

An early adopter of hemp, Barb was first in line to try CBD products when they first entered the sustainable living scene. A master gardener with twenty years' experience growing medicinal herbs and spices, she's also a recognized leader in the online homestead community, owner of the popular home and garden website RuralMom.com. She loves empowering others, including helping them to grow herbal remedies and embrace the cannabis culture.

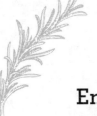

Endnotes

1   Centers for Disease Control and Prevention (CDC), "Unhealthy Sleep-Related Behaviors—12 States, 2009," *MMWR Morbidity and Mortality Weekly Report* 60 no. 8 (2011): 233–238, https://pubmed.ncbi.nlm.nih.gov/21368738/.

2   "BCBS Health Index," BlueCross BlueShield, last modified March 6, 2019 https://bcbs.com/the-health-of-america/health-index.

3   "Chronic Diseases in America," Centers for Disease Control and Prevention (CDC), National Center for Chronic Disease Prevention and Health Promotion (NCCDPHP), last reviewed October 23, 2019, https://www.cdc.gov/chronicdisease/resources/infographic/chronic-diseases.htm.

4   M. Michael Brady, "Viking Ship Cannabis Conundrum," *Norwegian American Weekly* (January 29, 2016), https://www.norwegianamerican.com/viking-ship-cannabis-conundrum/.

5   Çatalhöyük Research Project, last reviewed October 14, 2020, http://www.catalhoyuk.com/.

6   *Herodotus: The Histories*, trans. A. D. Godley (Cambridge. Harvard University Press, 1920). Hdt. 4.75, http://www.perseus.tufts.edu/hopper/text?doc=Perseus:text:1999.01.0126:book=4:chapter=75.

7   Epidiolex home page, https://www.epidiolex.com/.

8   R. L. Hawks and C. N. Chiang, eds., *Urine Testing for Drugs of Abuse* (Bethesda, MD: National Institute on Drug Abuse, National Institutes of Health), http://www.drugabuse.gov/pdf/monographs/73.pdf 1986.

9   Renée Johnson, "Hemp as an Agricultural Commodity," Congressional Research Service report, June 22, 2018, https://fas.org/sgp/crs/misc/RL32725.pdf.

10 "America's Founding Documents: The Declaration of Independence," National Archives, https://www.archives.gov/founding-docs/declaration

11 "Levi's Wellthread X Outerknown Present Cottonized Hemp," Levi's, March 4, 2019, https://www.levi.com/US/en_US/blog/article/levis-wellthread-x-outerknown-present-cottonized-hemp/

12 "Hemp," Patagonia, https://www.patagonia.com/our-footprint/hemp.html

13 "Sustainability at TOMS," TOMS, https://www.toms.com/environment.

14 Johns Hopkins Medicine "Some CBD Products May Yield Cannabis-Positive Urine Drug Tests," *ScienceDaily* (November 4, 2019), http://www.sciencedaily.com/releases/2019/11/191104141650.htm.

15 National Academies of Sciences, Engineering, and Medicine; Health and Medicine Division; Board on Population Health and Public Health Practice; Committee on the Health Effects of Marijuana: An Evidence Review and Research Agenda "Therapeutic Effects of Cannabis and Cannabinoids," *The Health Effects of Cannabis and Cannabinoids: The Current State of Evidence and Recommendations for Research.* (Washington DC: National Academies Press, 2017). 85–140 https://www.ncbi.nlm.nih.gov/books/NBK425767.

16 Shenglong Zou and Ujendra Kumar "Cannabinoid Receptors and the Endocannabinoid System: Signaling and Function in the Central Nervous System," *International Journal of Molecular Sciences* 19, no. 3 (March 2018): 833, https://doi.org/10.3390/ijms19030833.

17 "Endovanilloids Putative Endogenous Ligands of transient receptor potential vanilloid 1 channels," Mario van der Stelt and Vincenzo Di Marzo, Endocannabinoid Research Group, Istituto di Chimica Biomolecolare, Consiglio Nazionale delle Ricerche, Pozzuoli, Italy, *European Journal of Biochemistry*, no. 271(February 2004): 1827–1834.https://febs.onlinelibrary.wiley.com/doi/pdf/10.1111/j.1432-1033.2004.04081.x

18 Shenglong Zou and Ujendra Kumar. "Cannabinoid Receptors and the Endocannabinoid System: Signaling and Function in the Central Nervous System," *International Journal of Molecular Sciences* 19, no. 3 (March 2018): 833, https://doi.org/10.3390/ijms19030833.

19 M. De Feo et al. "Anti-Inflammatory and Anti-Nociceptive Effects of Cocoa: A Review on Future Perspectives in Treatment of Pain," *Pain and Therapy* 9 (2020): 231–240, https://doi.org/10.1007/s40122-020-00165-5. https://link.springer.com/article/10.1007/s40122-020-00165-5#citeas

20 Matthias B. Schulze. "Dietary Pattern, Inflammation, and Incidence of Type 2 Diabetes in Women," *The American Journal of Clinical Nutrition* 82, no. 3 (September 2005): 675–684, https://doi.org/10.1093/ajcn/82.3.675.

21 Benjamin Jowett *1892 The Dialogues of Plato: Charmides, or Temperance by Plato*, 3rd ed. (London: Oxford University Press, 2018). http://classics.mit.edu/Plato/charmides.html.

22 Kerstin Iffland and Franjo Grotenhermen "An Update on Safety and Side Effects of Cannabidiol: A Review of Clinical Data and Relevant Animal Studies," *Cannabis and Cannabinoid Research* 2, no. 1 (June 1, 2017): 139–154 doi:10.1089/can.2016.0034.

23 WHO Expert Committee on Drug Dependence. Fortieth Report, The World Health Organization (WHO), WHO Technical Report Series, No. 1013, 2018 https://apps.who.int/iris/bitstream/handle/10665/279948/9789241210225-eng.pdf

24 World Health Organization (WHO) "Cannabidiol (CBD) Critical Review Report." Expert Committee on Drug Dependence Fortieth Meeting (Geneva, CH: June 4–7, 2018). https://www.who.int/medicines/access/controlled-substances/WHOCBDReportMay2018-2.pdf?ua=1

25 Kerstin Iffland and Franjo Grotenhermen "An Update on Safety and Side Effects of Cannabidiol: A Review of Clinical Data and Relevant Animal Studies," *Cannabis and Cannabinoid Research* 2, no. 1 (June 1, 2017): 139–154 https: doi.org/10.1089/can.2016.0034

26 Juan Pablo Prestifilippo et al. "Inhibition of Salivary Secretion by Activation of Cannabinoid Receptors," Experimental Biology and Medicine 231, no. 8 (September 1, 2006): 1421–1429 https//:doi.org/10.1177/153537020623100816.

27 Khalid A. Jadoon, Garry D. Tan, and Saoirse E. O'Sullivan "A Single Dose of Cannabidiol Reduces Blood Pressure in Healthy Volunteers in a Randomized Crossover Study," *JCI Insight* 2, no. 12 e93760 (June 15, 2017), https//:doi.org/10.1172/jci.insight.93760.

28 U.S. Food and Drug Administration. "What You Need to Know (And What We're Working to Find Out) About Products Containing Cannabis or Cannabis-derived Compounds, Including CBD. Content current as of March 2020. https://www.fda.gov/consumers/consumer-updates/what-you-need-know-and-what-were-working-find-out-about-products-containing-cannabis-or-cannabis.

29 Centers for Disease Control and Prevention "Therapeutic Benefits," last reviewed January 2, 2018. https://www.cdc.gov/marijuana/nas/therapeutic-benefits.html.

30 Jürg Gertsch et al. "Beta-Caryophyllene Is a Dietary Cannabinoid," *Proceedings of the National Academy of Sciences of the United States of America* 105, no. 26 (2008): 9099–104 https://www.ncbi.nlm.nih.gov/pmc/articles/PMC2449371/

31 Amazon Seller Central. "Restricted Products. accessed June 25, 2020. https://sellercentral.amazon.com/gp/help/external/200164330.

32 Marcel O. Bonn-Miller et al. "Labeling Accuracy of Cannabidiol Extracts Sold Online," *JAMA* 318, no. 17 (2017): 1708–1709, https://jamanetwork.com/journals/jama/fullarticle/2661569

33 National Center For Complementary and Integrated Health, US Department of Health and Human Services, National Institute of Health "Melatonin: What You Need To Know", last reviewed October 2019, https://www.nccih.nih.gov/health/melatonin-what-you-need-to-know.

34 International Organization for Standardization. "ISO/IEC 17025:2005 General Requirements for the Competence of Testing and Calibration Laboratories," accessed June 25, 2020, https://www.iso.org/standard/39883.html.

35 Merriam-Webster Dictionary, "herbal medicine," accessed September 6, 2020, https://www.merriam-webster.com/dictionary/herbalmedicine.

36 University of Minnesota, "High Fat Foods Can Increase Oral Cannabidiol Absorption into the Body," *ScienceDaily* (August 13, 2019), www.sciencedaily.com/releases/2019/08/190813130426.htm.

37 Congress.GOV, "H.R.5587 To Amend the Federal Food, Drug, and Cosmetic Act with Respect to the Regulation of Hemp-Derived Cannabidiol and Hemp-Derived Cannabidiol Containing Substances, sponsor Rep. Peterson, Collin C. [D-MN-7]." (Introduced January 13, 20200, https://www.congress.gov/bill/116th-congress/house-bill/5587.

38 H.R. 8179—Hemp and Hemp-Derived CBD Consumer Protection and Market Stabilization Act of 2020, sponsor Rep. Shrader, Kurt [D-OR-5]. (Introduced September 24, 2020). https://www.congress.gov/bill/116th-congress/house-bill/8179

39 John McPartland and Ethan Russo "Cannabis and Cannabis Extracts: Greater Than the Sum of Their Parts?" *Journal of Cannabis Therapeutics* 1 (2001) 103–132. https://doi.org/10.1300/J175v01n03_08.

40 S. Nikfar and A. F. Behboudi, "Limonene," in *Encyclopedia of Toxicology* (3rd ed.), ed. P. Wexler (New York: Elsevier, 2014), 78–82. *ScienceDirect.* https://www.sciencedirect.com/topics/pharmacology-toxicology-and-pharmaceutical-science/limonene

41 USDA Agricultural Marketing Service,The Organic Seal, "How is Use of the USDA Organic Seal Protected?" Accessed June 20, 2020 https://www.ams.usda.gov/rules-regulations/organic/organic-seal

42 Fair Trade Certified, "Why Fair Trade?" accessed September 13, 2020, https://www.fairtradecertified.org/why-fair-trade

43 Regenerative Organic Certified home page, accessed September 6, 2020, https://regenorganic.org/

44 M. C. Cornelis et al., "Metabolomic Response to Coffee Consumption: Application to a Three-Stage Clinical Trial, *Journal of Internal Medicine* 283, no. 6 (February 12, 2018): 544–557, https://onlinelibrary.wiley.com/doi/abs/10.1111/joim.12737

45 D. C. Hammell, et al. "Transdermal Cannabidiol Reduces Inflammation and Pain-Related Behaviours in a Rat Model of Arthritis," *European Journal of Pain* 20, no. 6 (October 30, 2015): 936–948, https://doi.org/10.1002/ejp.818

46 Natashia Bruni, "Cannabinoid Delivery Systems for Pain and Inflammation Treatment," *Molecules* 23, no. 10 (September 27, 2018): 2478. https://doi.org/10.3390/molecules23102478

47 Office of Disease Prevention and Health Promotion (ODPHP), "Oral Health," accessed June 20, 2020, http://www.healthypeople.gov/2020/topics-objectives/topic/oral-health.

48 Division of Oral Health, National Center for Chronic Disease Prevention and Health Promotion, Centers for Disease Control and Prevention (CBC), "Periodontal Disease," last reviewed, July 10, 2013, https://www.cdc.gov/oralhealth/conditions/periodontal-disease.html

49 V. Stahl and K. Vasudevan "Comparison of Efficacy of Cannabinoids versus Commercial Oral Care Products in Reducing Bacterial Content from Dental Plaque: A Preliminary Observation," *Cureus* 12, no. 1 (January 29, 2020): e6809, https://doi.org/10.7759/cureus.6809

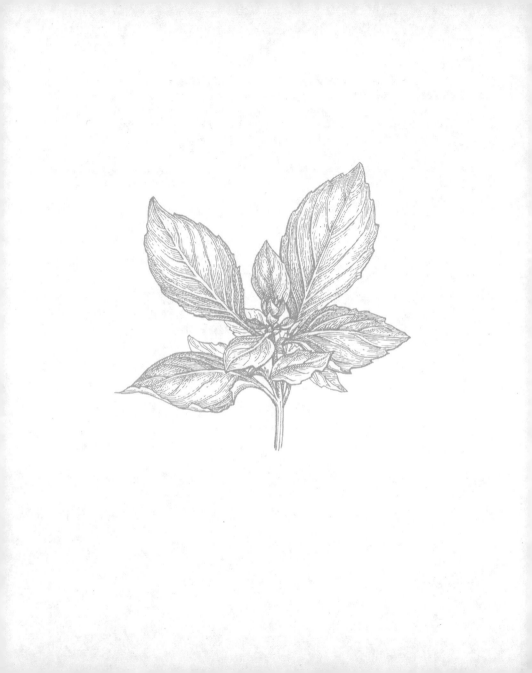